\\

SURVIVING CORONAVIRUS

How We Can Survive the Greatest Threat to Humanity since the Atom Bomb

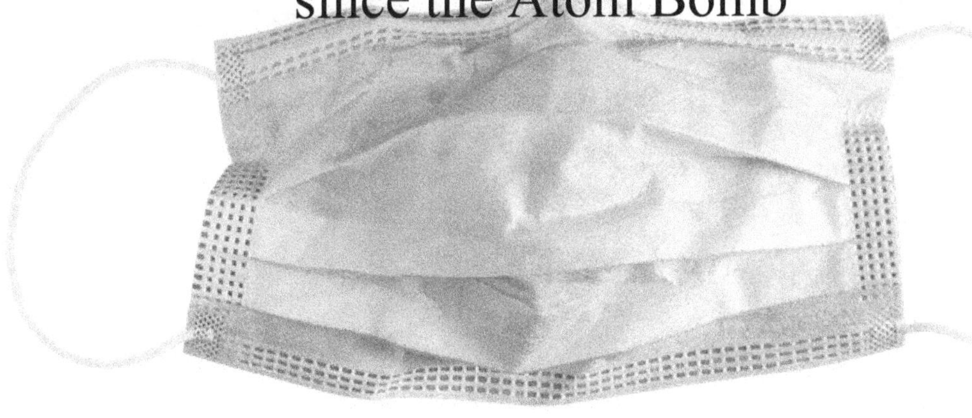

Garrett Bird, J.C. Harper, S. Lopin John, and Illia Rite

Multiple passages within this book are directly quoted from their respective sources. All sources are available in the Annotated Bibliography.

Cover Photos are property of Chatham House (Bombing of Hiroshima, Japan, 1945) and RawPixel (Surgical Facemask), 2020.

Surviving Coronavirus

How We Can Survive the Greatest Threat to Humanity since the Atom Bomb

By Garrett Bird, J.C. Harper, Illia Rite, and S. Lopin John

For our Fathers, lost before their times.

TABLE OF CONTENTS

Chapter 1

UNDERSTANDING THE MODERN BUBONIC PLAGUE:

How COVID-19 Swept the World

In 1945, at the end of the Second World War, the United States of America dropped two nuclear weapons on Imperial Japan—one on the city of Hiroshima, the other on the city of Nagasaki. The devastation created by these weapons was incalculable—their impact evaporated human beings, burned buildings, levelled mountains, and scorched the Earth. Hundreds of thousands of people were killed, either by the initial blast or in the irradiated fallout that lingered in the coming months and years.

The coming of the atomic bomb heralded a new chapter in mankind's history: one in which humanity held the tools for its own total destruction, one in which millions of lives could be extinguished by a single weapon. The sheer magnitude of the destruction brought on by the atom bomb brought one if its creators, nuclear scientist J. Robert Oppenheimer, to quote Hindu scripture on the power of gods: "Now I am become Death, the destroyer of worlds."

However, this was not the first time in human history that one single force held the power to wipe our species off the face of the planet.

Long before the Atom Bomb, there was the Plague.

The Justinian Plague

The first Plague was an outbreak of a disease called the "Bubonic Plague," which was transmitted through flea bites, caused horrible external and internal damage to the human body, and often proved fatal for its victims. This Bubonic Plague originated in southern Europe during the 6th century CE, during the reign of Byzantine (East Roman) Emperor Justinian I—for this reason, this specific pandemic is referred to as the Justinian Plague. While the Justinian Plague did not reach as far as subsequent pandemics, its outcome was still devastating: 30-50 million people, approximately half of Europe's population, were killed, and the plague spread into Persia and the surrounding territories in western Asia (Encyclopaedia Britannica, 2020).

Scientific and medical understanding of the disease at the time was incredibly limited, so hygienic preventative solutions and basic treatment were essentially nonexistent. We can speculate that the reason that this initial outbreak did not spread further was by simple limitations on traveling for victims. Trading and warfare within the Mediterranean region slowed to a crawl as a result of the Justinian Plague—this was also aided by the recent fall of the (Western) Roman Empire, which had been the central political and military power in the region before the 6th century. The Byzantine Empire, while powerful, did not have near the political influence or trading network of its predecessor.

As a result, the Justinian Plague remained mostly contained to the region of its origin.

The serendipity of this containment would not remain true for the second Plague.

The Black Death

The second Plague was yet another outbreak of the Bubonic Plague, but its effects reached even further. Emerging in the 14th century, the second pandemic, known colloquially as the "Black Death" because of the discoloration of bodily liquids brought on by the disease, originated in Central Asia and travelled along the Silk Road trading route back to Europe. Ravaging Europe, Asia, and much of North Africa, the second Plague proved even more catastrophic than the first. Within the duration of the pandemic, between 70 million and 200 million people, about a third of the total human population of Earth at the time, were killed (Encyclopaedia Britannica, 2020).

As with the first Plague, the second Plague was not medically well understood at the time. The famous "plague doctor" clothing, with goggled eyes and long noses, betrayed the idea that the Bubonic Plague was transmitted through breathing the air of its victims.

Hygienic preventative procedures to stop the spread of the disease, such as consistent bathing, handwashing, the disposal of corpses far away from drinking-water supplies, and the disposal and/or washing of clothing of Bubonic Plague victims, were not commonplace or consistent across Europe, Asia, or Africa.

In addition, the Silk Road which proved a boon to trade and travel between Europe and Asia made transmission of the Bubonic Plague all the easier than it was during the first outbreak some 800 years prior. The cessation of this trading came slower than it did in the 6th century, and consequently, the disease was able to spread further and faster.

The coincidence of medical misinformation and continued international travel brought about the nigh-apocalyptic event that remains the mostly deadly pandemic in human history. To date, no other disease has killed as large of a percentage of the human population as the second outbreak of Bubonic Plague.

But these conditions - medical misinformation and extensive international travel - would prove to be the root for the worst pandemics to come.

The Spanish Flu

The next terrible pandemic to analyze is an outbreak of influenza (also known as the common flu) that mutated into a more aggressive strain referred to as H1N1 in 1918, at the end of the First World War (Encyclopaedia Britannica 2020). You may recognize "H1N1" as being the same strand of influenza that would become referred to as "Swine Flu" in 2009, which we will discuss in the next section.

This outbreak originated somewhere around the middle of Europe in the vicinity of Poland in 1918. While medicine and our understanding of diseases had evolved far beyond where we were in the Middle Ages, the First World War had created a very specific set of circumstances that allowed for the proliferation of the virus across Europe and the United States.

First, given the notorious early use of "modern" artillery (machine guns, ballistic weapons, landmines, etc.) and chemical warfare, many people in Europe were already in compromised health— many were dealing with open wounds, missing limbs, or otherwise compromised respiratory systems. The brutality of the conflict, especially in trenches, meant that much of Europe remained in unsanitary conditions with people forced to remain closed in together in tight spaces, either moving from battlefield to battlefield or fleeing battles as they approached people's homes.

Second, the global nature of the Great War meant that soldiers were in transit all over the world, consistently, for the years-long duration of the conflict. This meant that all of the infected soldiers who had been in middle-Europe would eventually make their way to their home countries, whether that be Germany, England, Italy, Russia, the United States, and so on.

With both of these factors, people in mid-Europe were at a very high risk of catching the virus and these high-risk people ended up traveling all over the world. Thus, the influenza strain spread and claimed 25-50 million victims (Encyclopaedia Britannica, 2020).

It's worth noting here that Spain, which had remained neutral in the conflict, was neither the source of the influenza strain nor a focus point for it—the name "Spanish Flu" was coined in American journalism as a way to smear Spain's reputation in retaliation for Spain remaining neutral in the first World War.

The Polio Pandemic

Polio, an acute viral infection of the nervous system that leaves its victims paralyzed or killed, has technically existed for thousands of years. However, given that polio specifically latches onto compromised or weak immune systems (such as those in children with pre-existing health conditions), polio didn't become a serious problem for humanity until medicine and hygiene became advanced enough to allow for people with compromised immune systems to advance out of infancy (Encyclopaedia Britannica, 2020). This meant that the disease only grew into a pandemic in the late 19th and early 20th century.

By the mid-20th century, tens of thousands of cases of polio were recorded every year. While the disease was not nearly as widespread or lethal as its predecessors, polio's aggressive threat to children proved to terrify the general populace of the era. Images of children left entirely quadriplegic or attached to "iron lung" breathing apparatuses served as reminders for parents to keep their children isolated in the warmer months, when the virus was known to be most easily proliferated.

Unlike these previous pandemics, the polio pandemic's end can be traced back to the actions of one man specifically: a scientist by the name of Jonas Salk. While Austrian scientists had isolated the polio virus at the beginning of the 20th century, Salk worked to develop a vaccine to immunize children from this virus. By 1955, Salk's vaccine was tested and approved for widespread circulation. The results speak for themselves: cases of polio dropped off exponentially.

Modern medicine was finally able to respond to a pandemic and prepare a shield to defend the populace from spreading it once more. By injecting a modified, inactive strain of the virus and ensuring that entire communities were vaccinated using this strain (thus establishing what is referred to as "herd immunity"), humanity had finally found a reliable way to stop viral pandemics.

The only issue that we should take note of in the case of polio is that the virus strain was discovered in 1908 and Salk didn't have a model for the vaccine until 1953—this means that 45 years passed before a vaccine could be developed. While medical science has certainly advanced since 1953 (and even more so since 1908), developing a vaccine for a constantly evolving and mutating virus can still take a considerable amount of time and ingenuity.

Swine Flu

Now we come to the modern era, with the emergence of a new strain of H1N1 influenza in 2009 known colloquially as "Swine Flu." This strain of influenza originated not in Europe or Asia but rather in a small town in Veracruz, Mexico. It was in this small town that a young boy suddenly collapsed and was found to have caught a strain of H1N1 with several

commonalities to strains of influenza that were known to affect pigs (Encyclopaedia

Britannica, 2020). It is worth noting, in this case, that the flu could not actually be

transmitted by living pigs or pig meat.

Instead, direct human contact led to over 600,000 cases globally. Within a few

months, though, isolation efforts and travel restrictions spurred on by the United Nations

contained the spread of the virus to limited populations in affected countries. In tandem

with the containment efforts was the efforts to create a vaccine: thanks again to concerted

efforts by multiple world governments, an initial vaccine was developed just 5 months after

the outbreak of the disease.

Thanks to these measures, the Swine Flu pandemic was stamped out by the end of

2009. Humanity proved that pandemics like this could be swept up and taken care of quickly

and efficiently if we restricted travel, quarantined affected populations, maintained good

hygiene and cooperated on vaccine development.

This brings us to the current predicament that we find ourselves in today.

The COVID-19 (Coronavirus-19) Pandemic

In late 2019, a particular strain of coronavirus (a type of virus that affects the

respiratory system in mammals) emerged in the Wuhan province of China. It is theorized

that this strain of virus came from the consumption of bats in the region, a practice similar to the consumption of certain types of rattlesnake in the state of Texas in the United States of America.

Reporting on the outbreak proved to be slow, as recognition of the dangers the virus posed only really began in early February of 2020. Given that China is one of the largest economic powers in the modern world, with a vast system of domestic and international travel, the virus spread globally incredibly quickly.

The international community's response to the pandemic, much like China's, was built off of incomplete information and international travel that was all too slowly stifled. While Swine Flu was quickly identified and (relatively) quickly contained, the delayed identification and often prolonged incubation period of the virus (Coronavirus-19 can lay dormant for two weeks in a host body before the host begins displaying symptoms) meant that efforts to contain the virus came too late and carriers of the virus were often free to walk around for weeks at a time, with yet no mandate for a facemask. The variable levels of hygienic standards (facemasks, self-isolation, etc.) around the globe has not helped these matters.

As of the writing of this book, over 26 million people have caught Coronavirus-19. Over 850,000 people have succumbed to it (World Meters, 2020).

This means that more than four times as many people have been killed by this virus than were killed by the atom bombs dropped in Nagasaki and Hiroshima.

While the numbers of Coronavirus-19 have yet to reach the level of desolation brought on by the Bubonic Plague or the total destruction threatened by total nuclear war, we have no definitive timeframe on when a vaccine will be available. The number of cases continues to grow all over the world, even in some countries where it was presumed to be all but stamped out. While the majority of victims have eventually recovered from the virus (with many retaining potentially life-long respiratory damage), no definitive cure for the virus has been discovered or proposed. As Coronavirus-19 continues to mutate, it's possible for people who have overcome the virus before to contract it yet again.

Like it or not, the age of the pandemic is upon us for the foreseeable future. And if we falter in our efforts to slow its spread (stopping all unnecessary international travel, following hygienic safety practices like social distancing, etc.), humankind may be forced to look back to this moment as the third and greatest Plague in all of history.

Chapter 2

HOW LIFE CHANGED:

Empty Streets and Silence

While China and a handful of other nations were taking drastic steps to contain the virus by late February and early March, the worldwide response to the Coronavirus-19 epidemic went into full effect by April of 2020.

For one of the first times in all of recorded human history, hundreds of nations on every human-inhabited continent closed their borders and shuttered their businesses.

While it may be difficult to grasp just how far-reaching and all-encompassing these changes were, we will do our best to illustrate here.

From very early in 2020 until as recently as August 2020 (shortly before the publication of this book), the World Health Organization (WHO), a subsidiary of the United Nations, has strongly been pushing for restrictions on international travel, with precautionary measures in place to ensure that those who have to travel are tested and quarantined as is necessary and recommendations for governments of all member nations to adhere to the same precautionary health principles (WHO, 2020). Both of these steps, slowing international travel and instituting basic guidelines for intra-state handling of victims of the virus, were designed with the intention of limiting the spread of and, eventually, totally eliminating Coronavirus-19.

Based on how the spread of the virus has been stifled by nations that followed the guidelines more stringently and restricted incoming travelers early on (such as the notable case of the Pacific Ocean island-nation of New Zealand), this strategy makes sense. The strategy is soundly dedicated to preventing the virus from being able to spread, both domestically and internationally.

The upshot of this is that international travel has, indeed, been severely limited all over the world. As of the writing of this chapter, 79 countries remain totally blocked from international travel, while 87 more have heavy restrictions on who can come in and out of the country and 26 more have mandatory quarantine periods for all incoming visitors (Booking.com, 2020).

States that currently have either stringent travel restrictions or forbid all international travel include (but are not limited to):

- United States of America

- Canada

- China

- Russia

- Japan

- Greenland

- Iceland

- France

- Germany

- Spain

- Egypt

- India

- Indonesia

- Laos

- Malaysia

- Ghana

- Kenya

- South Africa

- Zimbabwe

- Argentina

- Chile

☐ Colombia

☐ Peru

☐ Venezuela

☐ Cuba

☐ Puerto Rico

☐ Denmark

☐ Belgium

☐ Ireland

☐ Italy

☐ Netherlands

☐ Norway

☐ Poland

☐ Sweden

☐ Israel

☐ Jordan

Movement between international borders, which had steadily been on the rise for decades, has suddenly slowed to a crawl. This was most apparently true with the plummeting value of airline and cruise stocks in early summer, which notoriously necessitated state intervention in multiple countries.

What this also means, of course, is that tourism has been drastically affected in multiple areas. While some locations opt to either remain open or open themselves to tourism prematurely, there is an overwhelming pattern of sudden subsequent outbreaks of the virus and massive closures and stringent quarantine procedures to compensate for the aforementioned outbreaks.

But tourism isn't the only aspect of everyday life that has drastically changed since the arrival of the virus. There are now massive closures, occupancy limits, and mask-restrictions for entering public places all over the world, including:

- Bars

- Grocery Stores

- Commercial Good Stores

- Medical Offices

- Shared Office Spaces

- Other Shared Closed Workspaces

- Restaurants

- Theaters

- Places of Worship

- Transit Hubs (e.g. Airports, bus stations, etc.)

This doesn't simply mean that these places are occupied by the same people, now with masks, from before the pandemic. This means that many of these places remain largely unoccupied at all, with huge swathes of stores, malls, or office buildings left mostly vacant for months on end.

Now, it's worth noting here that the internal quarantine/self-isolation restrictions have varied from country to country. In some larger, more fractious countries like the United States of America, where provincial governments divided by state and region hold considerable influence over the governing of their own respective areas, the restrictions have even varied on a regional level (As an example, New York and Hawaii, two traditional hubs for tourism in the USA, have much more stringent bans and quarantine periods for anyone wishing to visit than many of their counterparts).

As a whole, however, there has been a consistent global trend towards public and personal isolation as a response to the virus. Streets from Los Angeles to Hong Kong find themselves emptier, night clubs from Toronto to Nairobi find themselves quieter; the bustling, busy world of the 21st century now lays asleep, dormant, waiting for this pandemic nightmare to end.

However, the sickness caused by the virus and the global limitations on sharing public space to contain the virus aren't the only issues that have been brought to bear. As with the airline example mentioned earlier, there have also been far reaching economic effects the world over.

The slowing or outright ban on tourism all over the world has led to untold numbers of people with either much less profit than before or, in the case of low level workers dependent on tourism-based employers, potentially no jobs whatsoever.

You'll note the amount of advertisements in the past few months from airlines, cruise lines, and even the governments of traditional tourist locations encouraging you to come back "when you're ready," meaning when the pandemic is over. These advertisements are largely created in panic, as many of these companies and regions have become reliant upon travel and tourism to survive.

And while these industries and their ability to profit/function have been profoundly impacted by this pandemic, their employees remain even more vulnerable.

Of course, this issue isn't true to the tourism industry alone. In the cases of restaurants, bars, night clubs, retail stores, and other locations that have either been forced to close by government ordinances or by a sheer lack of customers, an untold number of workers have either been placed on some form of furlough or have suddenly found themselves unemployed. In some particularly egregious cases, the businesses in question either fold financially and become unable to pay for the unemployment benefits of their former employees or, far less ethically, the businesses in question retain workers on "furlough" without pay or expectation of providing more hours anytime soon, restricting their employees' ability to get any kind of living income or unemployment benefits.

This is especially a problem because not every country has provided economic stimulus/support to their citizens who have found themselves economically displaced by the pandemic.

As a result, we can see that the pandemic has caused a fourfold problem the world over:

1. People are either getting sick or are at great risk of getting sick from a disease that can have severe effects on the human body if not treated in due time

2. International travel and domestic commerce have been forced to slow to a crawl, resulting in a general sense of isolation that will likely have ongoing psychological consequences for every human living through it

3. This decrease in commerce and travel has caused an international glut in enterprise and economic growth, meaning that many industries are undergoing varying degrees of lost profits while relying on government subsidization to avoid bankruptcy

4. Multiple workers all around the world have found themselves suddenly lacking an income, meaning that they are now at risk of being unable to

afford their daily needs AND unable to afford the basic safety precautions to prevent the virus from spreading

Compounding these issues is the reality that at the moment, multiple private companies, travel-based and otherwise, are relying on government subsidization to stay afloat.

This is the primary justification that a number of world leaders have given for reducing and removing quarantine restrictions: if we retain these restrictions for too long, the economic impact on these companies will result in massive profit losses, lay-offs, bankruptcies, and, eventually, another global economic crash similar to the one that occurred in 2008.

The opposing viewpoint provided by most other world leaders is that while this may cause an economic downturn in the short term, the long-term effects of removing self-isolation/quarantine restrictions for Coronavirus-19 would be catastrophic. While the continued reliance on subsidization may cause a number of companies to face severe financial trouble in the near future, removing restrictions will almost inevitably result in a domino effect that would cause something akin to a second Great Depression.

The chain of events caused by the removal of safety restrictions are speculated to roughly be as follows:

THE WORST-CASE SCENARIO

1. Those infected by the virus will spread the virus in public spaces

2. The sheer amount of infected people will overwhelm the medical system, meaning that governments all over the world will be unable to keep up with testing and treatment

3. Deaths in medical facilities, either from the virus or from cases where there wasn't enough medical staff to handle all of the patients, will increase exponentially

4. The massive increase in deaths will result in a greater global panic, resulting in a complete collapse in consumer confidence in the market

5. A similar or worse glut in travel, tourism, and discretionary spending will occur, resulting in even more layoffs and even more corporate profit losses

6. More and more people will become sick or gain family members that are sick, resulting in households losing their income either due to the earners being sick or the earners being laid off due to the economic downturn

7. The worsening health of the general public, the large amount of lay-offs that will occur, and the lowered confidence in the economy will all feed on one another and make the situation even worse than it already is, ending in millions of people infected with Coronavirus-19 and the global economy in shambles.

Based on the disproportionate amount of governments that maintain their restrictions and precautions (see the list at the beginning of this chapter for a sample), it seems clear the worst-case scenario is incredibly unlikely to ever happen.

But that does mean that those familiar facemasks and emptier public spaces are here to stay for the foreseeable future.

That is why the rest of this book is dedicated to plotting out how to live with this new world we find ourselves in.

Chapter 3

MAKING PEACE IN YOUR MIND:

Techniques to Calm your Nerves

Stress is a vital part of the human experience. Afterall, stress originates in primitive times, when our hunter-gatherer ancestors relied on their fight-or-flight instincts in order to survive dangerous confrontations with violent animals and other natural threats. In that way, stress is a great motivator: under the right circumstances, that "positive" stress can help heighten your senses and give you the boost in energy to undertake difficult tasks.

However, too much stress is a problem. An unhealthy level of stress (which we'll call "negative stress") can ruin your ability to concentrate, bypassing all the benefits of the fight-or-flight reaction. Going even further, negative stress can cause headaches, high blood pressure, depressive or suicidal episodes, anxiety attacks, nervous breakdowns, and more.

The spread of the Coronavirus around the planet has, on average, produced far more negative stress than positive stress. According to the United States' Center for Disease Prevention and Control (CDC), the following are common symptoms of negative stress caused by the outbreak and constant observation of COVID-19:

- Fear and worry about your own health and the health of your loved ones, your financial situation or job, or loss of support services you rely on.

- Changes in sleep or eating patterns.

- Difficulty sleeping or concentrating.

- Worsening of chronic health problems.

- Worsening of mental health conditions.

- Increased use of tobacco, and/or alcohol and other substances. (CDC, 2020)

There are other symptoms that may arise as a result of this stress, of course, but these remain the most common. Similarly, the CDC has also reported that specific parties are more likely to be negatively affected by these symptoms. While it's true that parties who are at a higher risk to contract COVID-19 (e.g. the elderly and those with pre-existing health conditions) are likely to have a higher level of stress than many of their peers, this isn't the only group of people that may be having difficulty in these times.

Parties likely to feel this stress also include:

- Children and teens.

- People caring for family members or loved ones.

- Frontline workers such as health care providers and first responders, retail clerks, and others.

- Essential workers who work in the food industry.

- People who have existing mental health conditions.

- People who use substances or have a substance use disorder.

- People who have lost their jobs, had their work hours reduced, or had other major changes to their employment.

- People who have disabilities or developmental delay.

- People who are socially isolated from others, including people who live alone, and people in rural or frontier areas.

- People in some racial and ethnic minority groups.

- People who do not have access to information in their primary language.

- People experiencing homelessness.

- People who live in congregate (group) settings. (CDC, 2020)

So what can be done about this? With a comprehensive cure and/or vaccine likely to take yet more months to be formulated, how are we supposed to cope with the reality of Coronavirus in our day-to-day life?

Well, the first step is hard, but very important:

Don't lose hope.

Humanity has survived Ice Ages, the Bubonic Plague, the Spanish Flu, two World Wars, and the Cold War. Our resiliency is nothing to be underestimated.

In addition, while it may appear as though our society is struggling to come together to take on this threat, it's important to remember that Food Banks, Charities, and Crowdfunding Organizers are working to make sure that we save as many people as we can. Despite early shortages, masks are now being distributed consistently internationally. We're gradually stopping the spread of the virus, slowly but surely, and we're going to make it through this. Do your best to remind yourself of this at least once a day.

The second step is just as hard as the first, and it's just as important:

Take care of yourself as best you can.

This doesn't mean overindulging in alcohol, cigarettes, or other abusive substances or practices! Dr. Smitha Bhandari, a specialist in adult and teen psychiatry, suggests overreliance on substances, activities (even innocuous ones like video games or exercise), or specific individuals are likely to worsen one's stress levels in the long-term (Bhandari, 2020).

What this does mean is that you should attempt to incorporate the following into your daily life:

- Keep a positive attitude.

- Accept that there are events that you cannot control.

- Be assertive instead of aggressive. Assert your feelings, opinions, or beliefs instead of becoming angry, defensive, or passive.

- Learn and practice relaxation techniques; try meditation, yoga, or tai-chi for stress management.

- Eat healthy, well-balanced meals.

- Exercise regularly. Your body can fight stress better when it is fit.

- Learn to manage your time more effectively.

- Set limits appropriately and learn to say no to requests that would create excessive stress in your life.

- Make time for hobbies, interests, and relaxation.

- Get enough rest and sleep. Your body needs time to recover from stressful events.

(Bhandari, 2020)

Dr. Bhandari's list may not be incredibly specific about the procedure for each one of these steps, but they're invaluable as first steps in understanding what benefits your mind and your body.

To reemphasize the introduction to this chapter, stress ties back to fight-or-flight instincts, which come from your body: in other words, your mental health is inexorably linked to your body's health and wellbeing. This means that physical actions, referred to in Dr. Bhandari's list as "relaxation techniques" and "exercise," can directly alter and improve your mental health, reducing your stress levels.

So what sort of relaxation techniques are available to you? Well, yoga and tai-chi (from India and China, respectively) are variations of slow, deliberate physical exercise meant to strengthen the body and mind. While in-person lessons for both of these will be difficult to organize in the coming future, there are countless videos available online that can provide instructions on how to utilize the techniques of both practices to improve your stress levels.

"Meditation," as Dr. Bhandari lists it, can be religious, strictly psychological, or both. Various forms of meditation can also be discovered through online tutorials, including the traditional cross-legged, closed-eyed form that has come to be stereotypically associated with the term. By medical definition, though, even the dominant Christian conception of prayer, with knees bent and hands folded together, can be considered a form of meditation.

Thus, when Dr. Bhandari suggests "meditation" as a method of stress-relief, you should be aware that religious prayer of any kind absolutely counts as "meditation" and provides all the potential benefits therein. If praying can you help you feel better spiritually, it can definitely help you feel better mentally.

All of these practices (yoga, tai-chi, meditation/prayer) cost nothing but time, and if you are suffering from excess stress and have the time to practice them, it may be worth trying each one to see what works for you.

Of course, if you are lacking in time due to other obligations, there are other steps to take. The first is to step back and look at your situation: are all of the "obligations" that you're undertaking truly necessary? As stated before, overindulgence in activities, even ones traditionally viewed as being leisurely, can have a negative effect on your mental health. Sometimes postponing extraneous activities or reducing the amount of time you spend on extraneous activities can be the key to improving your mental health.

Maintaining connections while establishing healthy boundaries to those relationships is paramount to taking care of your mental health, and sometimes, communicating in relationships can feel more "obligatory" and stressful than they do refreshing or relaxing.

If you find that your obligations are caused by your relationships with others and you feel as though this is putting strain on your mental health, refer on ahead to Chapter 4 about remote communication (to reduce travel time for relatives) and/or Chapter 6 about negotiating boundaries and relationships with loved ones (whom you may now be involuntarily spending more time with).

If the obligations that you're undertaking now are directly tied to your financial stability, it may seem impossible to step out of them to get time to breathe. If you're suffering because you're in an economically endangered situation (wherein you lack confidence that you have the finances necessary to sustain you and/or your family), refer on ahead to Chapter 7 about attaining/maintaining financial solvency. Financial worries translate to worries for the bodily health of you and/or your loved ones, so they should be addressed just as seriously.

If you don't have the time for these physical relaxation techniques, or if they just don't work for you, don't give up! There are still other methods of relaxation and stress-relief available to you.

Aside from those techniques mentioned above, the CDC also strongly recommends that you take breaks from watching or reading the news (CDC, 2020). While it's important to stay informed about the outbreak and the dangers within your area, an endless stream of bad news will only serve to make you more worried or upset. At this point, you may not even be able to retain the excess information; all that will remain is that lingering sense of worry. Turn off the screens and put down the newspapers when you need to.

A simple change in your home or apartment can also make a world of difference to making your mind feel that little bit clearer. If you've been letting certain household tasks (like washing the dishes, cleaning the laundry, or organizing your common living space) build up over the last few months, it may be time to stop procrastinating and complete them.

After all, a dirty, cluttered, unorganized living space may only further increase your stress if you're stuck there all the time. Even if you're not able to safely invite guests over, there's no reason to force yourself to live in unnecessary discomfort. Your environment contributes to your bodily comfort, and as stated before, your bodily comfort directly contributes to your mental health. A nice, clean bed/couch/futon to sit on while eating food on a nice, clean dish can make a world of difference after a stressful day.

There are other changes that you can make to your environment that can help alleviate stress, as well.

Is there a particular smell that you enjoy? Or is there simply a smell that you've grown tired or sick of in your own home? It may be worthwhile to invest in getting some candles or electronic air-fresheners-- your olfactory sensors in your brain will likely welcome the change.

The same goes for the audio in your environment-- listening to music that you enjoy can certainly provide some amount of comfort, and now is the perfect time to discover other works that musicians or bands that you like may have created or been influenced by. Expand the playlist for your speakers or headphones and you just might find that your old bad mood will be singing a brand new tune!

And there's no need to simply stop there with audio-- you can also experiment with Autonomous Sensory Meridian Response (ASMR) sounds. These can range from the calls of seagulls and warm beach winds, to the rhythmic tapping of raindrops on a window, to less conventionally relaxing soundscapes like those you may find in a bar or party. Whatever sounds you may be missing, lacking, or needing right now can be simulated with a simple, free search on YouTube-- utilize the tools available to you to find the sounds that work for you!

Naturally, you're probably thinking you may not just want to clean your space, you may want to get a change of scenery all together. During a pandemic, your options are limited, but much like a theater stage, your home can look very different from other perspectives and with the slightest of changes. If you have access to more than one room in your home, consider spending time varied between different rooms at different times of day; if you spend time working in your living room, for instance, consider working in your bedroom or your kitchen, just to switch things up. If you have the more limited space of a studio apartment, shared or not, it may be worth your time to experiment with rearranging the furniture within your allotted space.

The human mind is built to recognize and track patterns, afterall; little changes in the daily routine can help break up those patterns to keep them from falling into monotony. A fresh new smell, some uplifting new music, and a bed moved sideways against the wall can make your whole world feel that little bit different or better to make things easier (Kitchener, 2020)!

Now, the rest of this book is dedicated to some other answers on how to handle various other aspects of living through this pandemic, including staying connected to loved ones (Chapter 4), finding new ways to keep having fun (Chapter 5), and how to manage your financial system despite dire circumstances (Chapter 7). Every chapter past this point could be construed as methods to reduce your stress regarding certain external stressors you may be facing right now regarding your relationships, recreation, and et cetera.

But don't forget that your mental health begins and ends with yourself. Only you can know if you're truly stable and/or happy. Do your best to take care of yourself utilizing any and all of the techniques in this chapter that work for you in a non-harmful, non-destructive, and non-addictive way.

Whatever you do, never forget that there's help available out there. If the stress of being cramped up in your home alone really is too much for you, never be afraid to call a loved one to talk.

And if the stress of this whole thing becomes just too much for you to handle on your own? That's okay. Know that it's not a sign of weakness to call a licensed medical professional, either within your healthcare system or through well-researched online sources like Better Help or Talk Space if you cannot afford healthcare, to see if you can get professional psychological help. To know your limitations is a mark of strength and bravery.

Remember: you're strong enough to have made it this far through the outbreak of COVID-19. You're strong enough to ask for whatever help you may need to make it through to the end.

Chapter 4

UNEARTHING CONNECTIONS ALL AROUND YOU:

Traversing Tools to Stay in Touch

Part of what makes us human is our need for other humans; who we are, how we define ourselves, how we measure our growth and goodness, is all dependent upon our relationship to other people.

In these times of self-isolation, it can be difficult to find and reinforce those connections. As the American Association of Retired Persons (AARP) notes, this is especially difficult for those who are elderly and/or living at home alone (Kassraie, 2020). It may be tempting, even, to break self-isolation and quarantine rules and simply act as though everything is fine.

But everything isn't fine; these standards and practices have been adopted internationally for a reason. It is important to avoid large gatherings, and, especially if you find your health or the health of your loved ones to be at heightened risk due to age or pre-existing conditions, it is important to limit all in-person contact outside of your home.

So what does that mean for that sense of longing, for that want to simply go out and meet other people?

Thankfully, we are not living in the times of the pandemics of the last millennium. We have access to a variety of technologies, methods, and resources in order to stay in touch, engage in mutually enjoyable activities, and even potentially meet new people to associate with.

Cellular devices of some variety, including the recently innovated smartphone, have become almost ubiquitous the world over. Nearly every adult owns a cellphone with access to phone calls, text-based messaging, and the world wide web. This means that it's always an option to schedule phone calls with your loved ones, or simply reach out to them through text messages to see how they're doing. There's no need to feel hesitant about doing so now, afterall: we're all in the same boat here in isolation. Your friends and loved ones will almost certainly welcome the contact (Kassraie, 2020).

In addition, it can be useful and enjoyable recreation to return to more traditional communication methods. Writing physical letters to loved ones, perhaps decorated with some personal touch or affection, can feel relaxing and authentic. If you've found yourself writing less letters over the past few years, then now may be the time to start writing them again; after all, even if you have phone calls with your friends every day, a nice little physical letter to remind them of your love certainly can't hurt.

The more sophisticated tools available to us in the modern day can also work wonders for keeping in touch. If your cellular device or computer has access to a web-camera (as most smartphones and laptops are), then you'll also have access to video calls.

There are a variety of programs that offer video call services for free: Skype, Zoom, Discord, Google Hangout, and Apple's Facetime are the most prominent examples of these. If a phone call can help alleviate that lack of connection, seeing your friends or loved ones' smiling faces over a video call can certainly bolster your mood.

Phone and video calls also offer you a variety of other options for engagement with your friends and loved ones. As *The Active Times* columnist Diamond Bridges writes, there's a whole world of activities to engage in utilizing phone and video calls, ranging from baking to game nights to movie nights to book clubs (Bridges, 2020). We'll elaborate on some of Bridges' points below.

Online Movie Nights

While it's not the same as watching something with someone else on a couch or in a pair of seats in a movie theater, phone and video calls offer you the experience of being able to synchronize with your friends and loved ones to enjoy a show or movie of your choosing.

With a variety of choices for streaming available to you, ranging from Netflix to Hulu to HBO Max to YouTube and Amazon Prime video and more, it's easier than ever to find movies you're interested in or your favorite movies of old and watch them with your loved ones. And, if you're going for a more classic approach in the style of cable, you can always check your cable channel schedule and set up a time for you and your friends or loved ones to sit down and watch an episode or movie as it premieres.

If you're utilizing video streaming or you're watching a home video (Blu-Ray, DVD, or even a VHS), all you need to do is countdown at the start of the video and hit play at the same time. Just like that, you can enjoy sharing commentary and/or the simple experience of enjoying a piece of media together!

Plus, the experience of watching it together means that you have something to discuss with your friends or loved ones afterwards, granting you a new topic of conversation and a new insight into your friends' or loved ones' opinions on films or shows!

Online Game Nights

You may or may not be familiar with video games that are typically played online, such as Mass-Multiplayer Online Roleplaying Games (MMORPGs) like *World of Warcraft*, or Multiplayer Online Battle Arena (MOBA) games like *League of Legends*, or Competitive Online Shooting games like *Call of Duty* or *Overwatch*. These games are typically played in the more traditional sense of skill and reflex based video games, with players using mouse-and-keyboard setups to put inputs into the games while utilizing headsets or other microphones to communicate with one another while playing.

While many find these games enjoyable, they're not for everyone.

If you're more accustomed or inclined towards traditional board or card games, no need to worry! These are also plentifully available online to play while on a phone or video call.

Popular applications and programs like *Words with Friends,* which offers you the ability to enjoy a game of *Scrabble* remotely, are bountiful online. You can enjoy card games like Gin Rummy or *Uno* through a variety of online sources. Through these same means, you can find simulators for board games like Chess, Checkers, *Trouble*, or *Monopoly*, and you can have fun with a handful of your friends for an evening almost as well as you could if you were gathered around a table!

You also don't have to be afraid of branching out into other non-traditional games. If you like trivia games like *Trivial Pursuit*, you may enjoy playing widely available games online like simulations of *Apples to Apples* or the more mature games like *Cards Against Humanity* or *JackBox.*

We remind you to be cautious in navigating games specifically, since there are a number of fraudulent or dubious websites out there offering them: it's recommended that you stick to trusted game providers like Steam to play them.

Once you're set up, though, you may discover whole new ways to have fun with your friends and loved ones.

Online Book Club

Not every activity that you utilize through video calls has to be undertaken simultaneously. Setting up a book club, which can meet at whatever level of frequency (once a week, twice a week, once month, etc.) that you're comfortable with can be a huge boon to keeping up with your literature-inclined friends. Just pick out a book for all of you to read and discuss your feelings on it upon returning to your meeting; whether you loved or hated the book in question, you'll certainly have something to talk about.

Book clubs can also be an excellent way to discover new books that you enjoy and bond with people over their deeper feelings on literature. A movie can be enjoyed all at once as an experience, but a book requires time to consume and mull over. Not only will you find that reading will make your time in self-isolation go by easier, it can provide you with an insight into your tastes and the tastes of those you connect with.

It can never hurt to exercise your critical thinking skills and keep your mind sharp!

Online Happy Hour

Taking some time to enjoy an alcoholic beverage or two with friends is a well-enjoyed pastime the world over. While bars may be closed or too dangerous to go to right now, you can always enjoy having a drink with your compatriots over a video call. Simply set up a time, preferably at a conventional after-work hour like 5 PM, ready some drinks of your preference, and enjoy. You can even ready some peanuts and snacks or a sports game to watch to add more authenticity to the experience!

Online Cooking or Baking

The joys of cooking and baking with someone can't be underestimated. The process of learning as you cook with someone else and the end result of having tasty food to eat are precious parts of being alive, after all.

While you can't hand a cup of flour through a computer screen, cooking along with someone else over a video call can still be immensely rewarding. Taking the time to pick out a recipe and both you and the person you're calling working to make the best of the recipe, side by side, is a fantastic way to build camaraderie. If one of you is more experienced with cooking than the other, then it can also be a fun teaching tool-- it's difficult to think of a better way to spend your time in self-isolation than working with your parent or friend to learn how to cook their signature dish.

Online Dinner Nights

We've discussed drinking, and we've discussed cooking: naturally, we can discuss eating.

There are few substitutes in life to the relaxation and enjoyment of eating a meal with friends and loved ones. Through a coordinated video call, you can enjoy that over a screen just as well. To make the experience more authentic, you can coordinate to make sure that you're even eating the same dish.

And don't be afraid to mix and match this idea with the happy hour, movie night, or cooking ideas; there's nothing wrong with getting creative and deciding to have a nice meal and watch a movie all in one night with your friends over video call!

Collaborative Journals or Story Projects

Collaborating in some kind of creative way is also a great way to keep up with others, whether it be writing a story together or simply writing a collaborative journal detailing your perspective on how things have been going around you. Programs like Google Documents allow you and your designated partner(s) to work on a document, add things, and make edits in real time.

Whether it's poetry, prose, or perspectives, if you and a loved one enjoy writing down your ideas, this always remains an option for you.

A Final Note: Social Media, Forums, and Group Chats

Finally, we come to the subject of meeting new people.

If you crave the feeling of going out and meeting new friends to interact with, don't fret while you're stuck at home: there's always options online for meeting new people you may enjoy talking to. There's always hobbyist groups and group-chats on Facebook, Twitter, and other social media websites. Hobbyist forums for subjects like knitting, at-home fix-em-up projects, exercise and more are littered all throughout the web; it's incredibly easy to create an account on any of them, and you can easily find more like-minded people with similar interests to talk to and, if you like them and feel comfortable enough, eventually get into phone or video calls with.

Now, as is the case with game installations online, we caution you to be careful when reaching out to make new friends: there is no reason that a new friend or hobbyist website or group should ask you for your Social Security Number or bank information, for instance. Always approach everyone new online with a measure of cautious optimism: surely there are other people looking to make friends just as much as you are, but you should be careful of anyone who may be looking to exploit you.

Once you can navigate this aspect of it, though, you may find several new, rewarding relationships. And remember: if you make new friends through these groups, forums, or social media websites, you can always spend time with them using some of the suggestions in this very chapter!

Chapter 5

FINDING ENTERTAINMENT EVERYDAY:
Exploring Ways to Keep Having Fun

At-home entertainment is nothing new to the average nine-to-fiver: looking forward to watching your favorite TV show or tuning into your choice of sports game after a hard day's work with a good meal and a seasonally temperature appropriate beverage is something the American public has grown fond of, even idolized.

However, now that the separation between work (at least with those lucky enough to maintain a job) and home has reached its absolute minimum, it's important to reanalyze how one spends their time engaging with media and diversion in general—one activity can tumble into another, and days can become time-warping blurs of either unremarkable or all too familiar activity. So, what solutions do we have available to combat mundanity in our daily lives, add richness and value to our minds and homes? Luckily for us, we have access to the hard work of others who've already taken this task upon themselves for the sake of their businesses and for folks like ourselves to utilize. But before we begin the process of searching through the endless stream of new media, let's talk a bit about what new and exciting categories are out there.

Ever since March 2020, things that may have once only been accessible in person at a venue (usually with lots of other people) have been digitized and made available online. Travel and Leisure magazine, for example, has compiled a list of 12 fantastic museums which have created virtual tours of their exhibits that you can peruse for free; Google search "Travel and Leisure digital tours" and that should lead to the article I'm referencing (https://www.travelandleisure.com/attractions/museums-galleries/museums-with-virtual-tours). One potentially annoying aspect of popular museums is that there are always crowds and noise at the most notable exhibits. Now, from the comfort of your own home, try perusing renowned works of art as if you had the whole museum to yourself.

If digitally traipsing around dusty old paintings and sculptures isn't your thing, perhaps try another newly digitized experience: on demand performances such as concerts, operas, plays, and musicals. Music artists and groups have begun hosting live concerts, streaming on sites like Youtube and Instagram. And while you're not exactly getting the full experience of being in a mosh pit with hundreds of other screaming fans, perhaps you'll get a preview of what your favorite musician will be like on stage when normalcy returns, plus no hearing damage! One of the larger events of this year when the critically acclaimed and typically sold out musical Hamilton began streaming on Disney+. Many more musicals and plays have also been recorded and made available online, all you have to do is figure out which platform they're being hosted on.

If you'd like to take a more educational approach to entertaining yourself, there are many different and wonderful online learning academies, some of which allow you to take extensive courses for free. Based on the subject, there are many different sites you may end up at, and finding the right site and course for you may require some personal research. If your tastes are more academic and you're working on a budget, one of the best and most easily accessible sites would be the Khan Academy (https://www.khanacademy.org/). They provide comprehensive courses ranging the gamut from college level math to personal finances.

If, now that you've been interfacing with a computer on the daily, you'd like to start learning to make your life easier by learning how to automate tasks through code, Codecadamy (https://www.codecademy.com/) has many more language specific courses than Khan and is also free (though with the option to pay monthly for premium support throughout your learning process). If you'd like to begin learning an art or some of the "softer" sciences (like cooking!), Udemy (https://www.udemy.com/) offers a very wide range of courses you can take. With Udemy, however, you'll be paying by the course, though some courses are offered for free.

Podcasts and books/audiobooks are also excellent options for self enrichment. There are all different types of podcasts ranging from comedy talk shows to weekly breakdowns of the latest in artificial intelligence. Websites like PodChaser (https://www.podchaser.com/) have lists and lists of the latest casts broken down by category, and can be an excellent resource for newbies. If you're the type of person who used to read for pleasure, but a busy life has made other plans for your downtime, audiobooks may be your saving grace. Now whenever your hands are busy and your mind is free, you can enjoy an escapist fantasy or gritty mystery—laundry will never be the same. Audible (https://www.audible.com/) has been a growing presence in the book community, and they feature a membership program where you're allotted credits per month which you can spend to purchase **any** book you'd like to listen to, one per credit—you can always purchase more credits or purchase books without either a membership or credits. When searching for the perfect book or audiobook, sites like GoodReads (https://www.goodreads.com/) have a plethora of wonderful reviewers who curate themed reading lists for your consideration.

Load up your latest podcast and put on an apron, because the next often overlooked and underappreciated activity could get messy. Cooking can be a fun, rewarding, and (hopefully) tasty venture that can add some literal spice to your life and turn doldrums into dol-yums. For the aspiring home chef there are countless food blogs and recipe sites, so sometimes a simple Google search of "stew recipes" can turn into an all out expedition. Google attempts to make this easier by posting the star rating of the recipe next to the link, but the best tip we can offer is, read the comments. There are always useful modifications and measurement adjustments posted by foodies that can elevate dishes to greater heights.

Also, don't stop with the first result you find, compare recipes and see where the differences are and if that makes sense to you. Also whether you're living alone or are the main food source for your family, as long as you've been to a supermarket in the last few months, you should have noticed that there have been food shortages and you may be wondering how to make canned beans and rice seem exciting. Sites like Supercook (https://www.supercook.com/) and RecipeLand (https://recipeland.com/) make finding interesting recipes by available ingredient a breeze.

And while those beans are bubbling away, now's the perfect time to enrich not just yourself but your living space with a little tidying up. Okay, so maybe not as fun as browsing the net for your next favorite book, but lack of hygiene and order can quickly become a silent stressor when you're spending your entire day in one environment. Additionally, in a world where we're trying to contain an extremely contagious virus, it'd be a good idea to sanitize your most public spaces if you're living in a group scenario or even just the hot zones if you live by yourself.

And speaking of hot zones and cooking, the kitchen sink is a particularly egregious breeding zone for bacteria, so perhaps a quick wash while you're in the mood to clean is a good idea. If you're the type of person who is having issues motivating yourself, there are a few applications which allow you to "gamify" your tasks. Habitica (https://habitica.com/) is a cute and easily accessible site which turns the mundane into the magical with its fantasy style: as you complete chores that you assign, you'll be increasing skills and levels for your character. Tying things back, a set of headphones will allow you to listen to your favorite audiobook even while vacuuming—from personal experience, we recommend cordless.

So now that we have all the pieces in place, let's talk about the one activity that has ascended to a high artform in this era of social-distancing and working from home: the perfect binge. If you're approaching this au naturale, hopefully we've provided enough tools in this chapter for you to plop down on the couch after a long day of enriching yourself, with your latest culinary masterpiece, in your nice neat and clean living space, put on your favorite show and just go to town—let the body set the limits and see just how deep that rabbit hole goes. If we're approaching this scientifically, however, it's important to set healthy, obtainable goals and parameters (though one's definition for either adjective may, and perhaps should, vary) and make sure you have, the show or set of movies you'll be watching.

First things first, you're going to want to settle on the show you'll be binging. If you're one of the few people who has yet to experience the information overload of streaming services such as Netflix, Hulu, or Amazon Prime you've probably made a good series of life choices. However, if you would like to dip your toes in now or if you are an individual who has indulged in the immediate gratification of on demand media, but now you're discovering that the content you're viewing has taken a turn to mediocrity, perhaps it's time to dig into the nitty gritty of finding new and interesting shows.

We should note that if you're just looking to find which streaming platform(s) have a show or movie that you've already selected, Google does an excellent job of making the search for that service quick and easy. Simply type the name of the media into their search engine and in the results, on the right hand side of the screen, you should see a side panel with a drop menu aptly named "All watch options". Simply click that text and you'll see which streaming platforms offer that media. But, if you've watched everything that you've been interested in so far and don't have a film critic friend who can recommend interesting television and movie options, there are alternatives to simply clicking on the next recommended from your streaming platform.

The most basic, and sometimes best, option is to simply search the internet for "movies/shows like <insert something you already like here>". There are a multitude of Internet forums and message boards with aficionados more than willing to express their opinion on what exactly you should be watching next. If you would instead like to track your progress through shows and be recommended new ones automatically (without the bias of your streaming platform) there are sites like Trakt (https://trakt.tv/) which act as a small scale social media platform allowing you to interact with other fans of the same show and brings you the latest information about new episodes and news regarding your favorites.

If you would like to quickly see what's fresh and new on the streaming markets, you can always head over to Rotten Tomatoes (https://www.rottentomatoes.com/). Famous for their aggregation of scores from both big name critics and regular viewers, Rotten Tomatoes is mostly known for their movie reviews. However, they are an equally valuable source for new info on premiering and returning shows, as well as offering ratings. Whatever your method—be it friend, algorithm, or review—make sure you have two or three shows/movie series selected in case you don't like your first choice.

Now that you've got your target in sight, it's time to construct your plan of attack! If you're doing a three episode mini-series, perhaps little planning is required: simply make sure you're comfy and hydrated, and just one-shot it. Most likely you'll have a series that goes a little longer than 3-4 hours, so how do we break it up? Hopefully if you're a desk worker (either at a business office or now from your home office), you're already making sure that you're moving around and diversifying what you're staring during the work day.

According to WebMD, you should be following the 20-20-20 rule when staring at a computer screen, that is to say, for every 20 minutes of screen time make sure to stare at something at least 20 feet away for at least 20 seconds.

Following that easy rule, as well as getting some quick and easy exercise during the day (skip to chapter 8 for some tips on that), will make it a lot less impactful on your body as you dive fearlessly, headfirst into a 176 hour series like *Star Trek: Deep Space 9*. As for how many hours you should be watching per day, that's really up to how much endurance and time you have, as well as your age.

For people ages 50 - 71, studies have shown that those who watch five or more hours of television per day have a 65% higher chance of developing mobility disabilities when compared to those who watched two or fewer hours of television. Does that mean that you can't occasionally have a full movie day if you're past 50? Of course not! The antidote prescribed from the same doctor who conducted one the studies, Dr. Loretta DiPietro, is to get up and move around once every 30 minutes, the results of which would phenomenally reduce the risk of mobility issues and heart disease. And for the young bucks and does reading, this doesn't give you the green light to sloth out with impunity. If you feel like you've been clocking in the hours on screens, be it smartphone or laptop, and not following the 20-20-20 rule, you're risking vision impairment later in life as well as a multitude of other developmental issues. So to summarize, set yourself up for success prior to your binge with exercise and screen etiquette, set realistic limits for how long you'll be viewing your series during the course of one day, break up your viewing party with intermittent marches to the restroom or at least standing up and taking a circuit of the couch.

If you're lucky enough to be quarantining with loved ones or friendly roommates, you've found the loophole through to the social part of social distancing, and your binge can become a binge party with food, commentary, and good spirits. However, if you're toughing out the virus alone, you might find it a bit challenging to watch hours and hours of media solo. Fortunately there are tools available that make creating online watching parties a facile task. Netflix Party (https://www.netflixparty.com/) is a great option if, quite obviously, your designated streaming content is available on Netflix. Downside is there is no voice/video to stay in contact with the other party members and so you will need a third party conferencing app (Discord, Skype, Zoom, Phone if you're desperate).

Similarly there are integrated "watch party" apps for both Hulu and Amazon prime, with similar downsides to Netflix Party, though Hulu Watch Party requires at minimum a No Ads subscription. If you're looking to stream from one account only, you can attempt a Zoom call and share screen from the host's computer. This will work for any streaming service, though the downside is it's highly reliant on the host's upload speeds, else everyone will be viewing sub-par quality. If hosting viewing parties is something that you take pride in and don't mind spending a bit of money, TwoSeven (https://twoseven.xyz/) offers syncronized viewing of almost every streaming platform available, and at just $3/month you're able to get the full package. There is some minor setup, subscribing to their patreon and getting everyone set up, but they offer video and voice in addition to a text-based messaging system. Lastly, if worse comes to worst, you can always just find a conferencing app and do the old countdown method: 3-2-1… watch!

By this point you should be fully capable of finding yourself comfy and settled on a couch or bed with a full stomach and snuggled up with whatever media you'd like to consume. Whether it's a nice new book you're listening to or reading, or you're engaging with some new and exciting enrichment content, life at home during this unprecedented pandemic need not be dull and grey. Enjoy every day to its fullest and *thrive*!

Chapter 6

MITIGATING CONFLICT AT HOME:

Easing the Stress of Constant Cohabitation

Whether you are an essential onsite worker, remote worker, or currently unemployed because of the pandemic, everyone is now spending exponentially more time with their family or housemates than ever before. While that can most certainly be a positive experience—getting to really enjoy extra quality time with those you cohabitate with—it can also cause certain stress and anxiety for those unused to it.

Everyone is adjusting to the new rules of life to help them stay safe, between wearing masks in public spaces to washing your hands when getting home, there are different emotional challenges that COVID-19 has presented for us all. It is important to be aware of your own mental health as well as that of those around you to make this part of the "New Normal" more navigable.

Living with Family

Quarantine has presented new challenges for families cohabitating, whether just parents and their children or having extended family staying as well, everyone is trying to demarcate their space in the home and work with having closer quarters than before.

Especially for parents whose children had just started an independent life off at college who are now coming back into the home, what is most important is open communication and higher empathy in these trying times. Everyone is working to adjust their routines and lives around what is currently available, and especially for members of the household who were more actively out of the house, there has been a learning curve for understanding what to do without avenues out of the house they could usually take.

For parents and adult children who had to fly back into the nest during these times, it's hard for the parents in that situation not to fall back into the old patterns of parenting and control they previously had over their child. The adult child, meanwhile, is probably battling different anxieties and frustrations from having been working towards a more independent life and now having to reorient themselves to being once again in their parent's household. It's important, therefore, to try to set ground rules for sharing the house, as well as "devising a contract for managing household responsibilities, like how a family will share the same bathroom, washer and dryer and refrigerator" (Halpert, 2020). These of course would need to be morphed to fit the living situation and responsibilities expected of each party, but it is a good start with this sort of foundation as well as an understanding of chores and a healthy respect for boundaries. Both parents and adult children will benefit from trying to understand each other's positions and hearing each other out to make the living situation between them as comfortable and supportive as possible.

As for assisting younger children who are adjusting to a huge change in their daily routine, it is important to monitor how they are feeling and see what is and isn't working for them in quarantine. Depending on the child and how social they were previously, they can be experiencing anxiety and stress from less time with schoolmates and no sleepovers with friends. However, during the switch to online schooling, there have been various positives and negatives for the e-learning for children. There are various studies that argue school's early startup time is not giving children the amount of sleep they need, so for some the extra rest and time that comes from not going physically to school has given them time for creative pursuits and activities with their family both physically and through the internet. When you find something that can help alleviate the stresses they are experiencing, to encourage them to balance that activity with their studies and give them reassurances in a very unsure time.

A parent knows their child best, so being aware of these things as well as their own mental health will allow for parents and children to understand each other. Childhood, in many ways, is now more free than it had been previously for kids, with less structured time being forced upon them by the busy American culture they were growing up in. Children are experiencing room to breathe in an unintended way, and have time for "trying new things, helping more, discovering new interests, spending more time outside and with family, and learning in new ways" (Clopton, 2020). While it is certainly a mixed bag, there is good evidence that the rigorously structured lives many kids led previously could use some rethinking after these months of quarantine. While it's good to keep children engaged and have activities for them, it is also good to allow them room to explore what interests them and who they are.

It's a small blessing that many children are now getting to do just that.

It may be difficult in this time for those who may have been more used to the pace of their relationships with their children being dictated by their jobs to adjust to this new intimacy, especially given that their expectations of what would've been good for them in childhood during a pandemic may clash with what their children actually want. Nevertheless, this is the time to learn, empathize, and negotiate how that time is spent. You may not think about COVID-19 24/7, but this moment is traumatic for all of us. Try to remember that and be especially empathetic to the infants, children, and young adults who may not be able to grapple with that yet.

Living with Roommates

Under normal circumstances, living with roommates can be a mixed bag. On the one hand, there is a lot of freedom and enjoyment that can be had sharing a space with another adult who assists with bills and does not necessarily require anything else of you. On the other hand, sharing a space with other adults means figuring out what is important about the living space for both you and them as well as negotiating space, schedules, and chores. This can be a big challenge under normal circumstances, and we are in very abnormal circumstances. For that reason, roommates now more than ever need to be communicating about their new needs for the space and their understanding of daily routines.

Especially if one or more of your roommates is now working remotely, this will require a negotiation of the space they occupy during their work hours and needs for that time. If they work a job with a large amount of meetings or time on the phone with coworkers or customers, this can mean the need for quiet in hours where it was not necessary before. If your roommate is an essential worker, this means they are out in the field facing the threat of COVID in the way a remote worker might not be. For them, understanding and empathy is highly necessary, but also devising of an agreement about what kind of hygienic requirements are needed for both of you to feel comfortable. Once again, open communication is key to maintaining a good living situation.

Another problem roommates will face is deciding how they are going to navigate Common spaces depending on their living situation. They may be sharing common laundry rooms, dining rooms, or kitchens with people they are not living with. Of course, if you can use these facilities only within your apartment and avoid them elsewhere, this is recommended. If not possible, though, remember to take measures to protect yourself and others. It is important to remember in hallways, laundry rooms, and other facilities used by people you are not rooming with, to maintain the Center for Disease Control and Prevention's (CDC) recommended 6 feet of distance and to bring your mask. Other recommendations by the CDC include:

- "People who are sick, their roommates, and those who have higher risk of severe illness from COVID-19 should eat or be fed in their room, if possible.

- Do not share dishes, drinking glasses, cups, or eating utensils. Non-disposable food service items used should be handled with gloves and washed with dish soap and hot water or in a dishwasher.

- Guidelines for doing laundry such as washing instructions and handling of dirty laundry should be posted.

- Sinks could be an infection source and should avoid placing toothbrushes directly on counter surfaces. Totes can be used for personal items so they do not touch the bathroom countertop" (CDC, 2020).

Remember to consider all of these things to keep yourself and your living mates healthy and happy. If they are unaware of these recommendations, informing them in your living contract can be a good way to reach an understanding on these matters. Trying to work along these guidelines and understanding each other in this trying time will be your greatest tools to avoid conflict.

Living with your Partner/Spouse

For those who are living together with just their significant other, there a both similar and different challenges to be overcome. There are many articles out there discussing the challenges that married couples are facing, but couples who have not tied the knot are not as widely discussed. Young couples between the ages of 18-24, however, do make up 9% of the couples living together, as opposed to the 7% of their age group that are married (Sassier, 2020). If you are a younger couple that just started cohabiting before the pandemic began or you've been living with your partner for a while, the new stresses of cohabiting during a pandemic are unfortunately. Many among their age group are being impacted by the widespread layoffs throughout the US, since they are not as senior in their fields and especially for those who earned college degrees and were newly entering the job market. Others are dealing with the changes to their college curriculum and new challenges for getting their degree.

In all these cases, young couples will need to pull together and communicate to make sure they are not stepping on each others toes. A relationship is always work, but hearing out your partner's daily ups and downs will be more important now than ever before.

While you may expect your partner to operate as they usually have because you crave that sense of stability, recognize that both of you will be undergoing at lot of emotional duress and change forced upon you by the circumstances. Where usually one partner might be able to shrug something off, they may now be unable to emotionally handle the same situation and shut down or explode outward. It's important to recognize when it is best to be together, and when it might be best to give your partner some space.

The range of emotions we are all going through are wide—there will be times you want to laugh hysterically and times you feel entirely hopeless.

These types of struggles can be voiced to your partner, but remember that no relationship is a substitute for professional help. Telehealth visits are now highly offered for various health needs, from clinical visits to therapy visits, and they should be explored if you ever feel there is so much that you cannot work it out with yourself and others. Being mindful of this, make sure that you are still monitoring the healthiness of your relationship. Recommend these same things to your partner if necessary, but also recognize that there are points to which unhealthiness can escalate to be harmful to yourself.

With the pandemic and sheltering in place being the norm, chances for domestic violence can go up, and it is important to recognize signs and never ignore it if the situation escalates to that between you or your partner. Stress over the situation is no excuse to be violent to loved ones and should be immediately dealt with, and domestic violence resources should be researched and reached out to.

Remember that from families to roommates to couples, everyone is going to have to be highly empathetic to those they are sharing space with. While there are benefits to not be quarantining alone, remember that everyone needs personal space and time to process and understand their emotions.

Work to understand each other, talk out what is necessary for everyone to feel comfortable, and remember to monitor your emotions and never let a situation where you are unsafe spiral out of control.

The world outside our homes may be uncontrollable in many ways, but we can work to mitigate the issues we experience within our own space. Afterall, as we've emphasized previously within this book, we're all in this together. Not one person on this planet is immune to the virus. Not one person on this planet is immune to the societal changes occurring as governments the world over prep us to attempt to contain it.

Your roommates, your friends, your parents, your grandparents, your siblings, your cousins, your children, your partner-- all of the people in your life are facing the same challenge right now.

Take a deep breath.

We can make it through this. Remind yourself and those you love of that truth through your actions every day.

Chapter 7

FINANCIAL MANAGEMENT IN CRISIS:

How to Maintain or Find Solvency

This health crisis we face is almost as dangerous to our wallets as it is to our lungs. The United States of America alone has seen record levels of unemployment, as an unprecedented amount of people are suddenly out of the job while their employers are forced to close for safety reasons. For many, even in places where businesses are reopening, the choice to remain unemployed makes the most sense when the alternative is being exposed to the virus and having to face the economic reality of the costs of paying for Coronavirus treatment.

Even people in relatively secure white-collar positions within corporations are seeing threats to their ongoing financial wellbeing, as corporations are now constantly reviewing what staff they need to keep on or how much of a reduction in pay is necessary to make up for lost profit, and as the stock market has become historically volatile and vulnerable to collapse as good and bad news trickles in.

Under these circumstances, it's completely understandable to be worried about your financial security. But don't lose hope. There are still things you can do to make sure that you and your family are secure.

In order to provide more focused explanations of specific financial situations, we'll be breaking this chapter into two halves: one for a situation where you do not have reliable income, and one for a situation where you do. While it's perfectly fine to skip to the section that applies to your current situation, we advise that it will be useful to read both in order to be prepared in case your situation becomes better (i.e. you find a source of reliable income) or if you find a friend or loved one without reliable income in need of advice on what to do.

If You Do Not Have Reliable Income: Securing Reliable Income

There are a variety of reasons that you may not have reliable income right now. Like many workers at "nonessential" jobs, you may have been laid off while your place of employment has been shut down due to current public health restrictions. Even if your place of business has reopened, as stated above, it's an understandable decision to forego returning to a service-based position when the risk of catching coronavirus and having to pay for treatment outweighs the amount of money you'd get by returning to work.

You may have had a job that you thought was stable, but got downsized and removed from your place of work so that your employer could "lean down" and avoid paying all of their employees.

You may not have had a job to beg with because you were a student, which means that you also likely haven't had the time to build up a job history.

If you find yourself in one of these circumstances or some variation thereof, where does that leave you?

A first important step would be to apply for your state's unemployment benefits (preferably online, as their phone lines are apparently swarmed and riddled with long waiting times). Losing employment, especially under these extenuating circumstances, is nothing to be ashamed of, and there's absolutely no shame in getting help from an apparatus built to help citizens in times of national and personal crisis.

It's possible, especially if you've recently graduated from college, that you won't qualify for unemployment due to a lack of established job history. What do you do in that case?

Well, the United States' Consumer Financial Protection Bureau (CFPB) has plenty of programs for coronavirus assistance available on their website, https://www.consumerfinance.gov/coronavirus/, ranging from programs to assist in mortgage payments to specific tax advice for parents and the elderly. The CFPB also has several details on its website for programs to assist in getting unemployment insurance and other financial assistance for veterans, recent students, and other protected classes of citizens (Consumer Financial Protection Bureau, 2020). If you find yourself in this precarious position in the first place, we would advise that you go to their website to see what help you may be eligible for.

In addition, the CARES Act, passed by the United States Congress in spring of 2020, allows for expanded opportunities for recent college graduates in the United States in particular (Kara, M. and Gentry, R. 2020). While this is based largely upon your having some form of previous job history, we would still highly advise that if you are a recent college graduate or know someone struggling after graduation, you should definitely research the CARES Act or your country's equivalent.

With all of this in mind, we understand that there are many people who out there who may have been unemployed before the Coronavirus epidemic and, having been unable to secure a job in the intervening time due to restrictions on hiring across the globe, are thus ineligible for any form of government assistance or unemployment payments. To any who may feel incredulous about the number of people in this circumstance, we urge compassion and an open mind: this type of circumstance often comes at the expense of people from impoverished families and/or people who have some form of disability (physical injury, physical illness, mental illness) that may inhibit their ability to be hired or keep a job.

If you are in this particular circumstance, where you are ineligible for unemployment benefits at this time and you have exhausted all other avenues for application, please don't give up hope.

If you suffer from a situation like this one, brought on by some form of illness or tragic event, you always have the option of utilizing a crowdfunding website, like KickStarter or Gofundme, to solicit funding from other citizens through social media such as Twitter or

Facebook to try to get more help in your situation. While it's by no means a sure-fire solution, it remains an ever-present option, if only for minor assistance.

Beyond that, we advise looking into all possible options for at-home employment. Whereas work-from-home occupations were once considered rare and difficult to come by before the epidemic, they are now rather commonplace: large telecommunication-based companies in particular, like HBO, Comcast, Netflix, and Verizon, are now hugely reliant on at-home employees providing easy-to-understand technical assistance to customers all over the globe. If you have access to a smartphone (and, preferably, a laptop or computer of some sort), you have a very good chance of finding employment with one of these call-help occupations. While telemarketing suffers from a less than wonderful reputation, this is also a field of employment that remains largely accessible with very few job or education requirements barring entry to anyone in need of income.

If these positions do not work for you, whether it's due to a lack of access to technology or due to the jobs not paying enough to support you and your family, we can advise that you review websites like Monster, Indeed, and LinkedIn to review any and all openings for jobs that allow work from home. We reiterate that at-home employment is the safest option at this time, which is why we must advocate for that avenue forward. Only take employment that does not allow for work-from-home if you find that it is absolutely, totally necessary.

However, if none of these options work for you, and you don't find yourself able to work right now for whatever physical or psychological reason, we highly encourage looking into community mutual aid programs. Many of them are listed online, and reaching out for help to people within your community for aid can be far more reliable and rewarding than relying on distant government entities or private crowdfunding websites.

And if you don't have a computer to look, don't worry: your local library, of which there are many all over the globe, should have computer access for you to use in order to seek out employment online.

Explore all avenues for help and employment, apply where you can, and keep on fighting to get that stream of income. We believe that you can do it, and that your friends and loved ones can do it, too, if we're all willing to lend a helping hand where we can.

If You Have Reliable Income: Managing Your Money Responsibly

If you have reliable income, either now or after following the steps in the above section, then we bid you congratulations: you're already in a pretty good position.

With that in mind, we also understand that there are two points of concern even in cases where you have reliable income:

1. "I don't think my income is enough to sustain me and my family." This is a concern for the present.

2. "I don't know how I should be managing savings and investments at this time." This is a concern for the future.

Let's begin by addressing the concerns for the present, concern about your income being insufficient to take care of you and your family.

To start, we must reiterate both the message of the previous section and the resources therein: it is not shameful to ask for help if you need it. Government programs, such as those to provide aid for parents, veterans, the disabled, and recently graduated students, are in place explicitly to help vulnerable people in a time of crisis. We are in a time of crisis, internationally and personally, so it's perfectly reasonable and respectable to apply for that assistance.

My aforementioned statements from the Consumer Financial Protection Bureau (CFPB) remain true: there are a variety of government programs to help ease your burden when it comes to mortgage payments, food stamps/vouchers, or student loan payments. We strongly encourage you to look into those programs that may be applicable to your situation, as their website is always readily available online.

Aside from receiving government assistance, just as was the case with seeking a source of consistent income, there are indeed steps that you can take to secure your financial security. To begin with, it will be useful for you to review all of the bills that you may be paying at this time and reviewing which aspects of monthly spending are strictly necessary. This isn't to say that you should cut yourself off from any and all forms of recreation in order to pay for necessities like rent and groceries, but rather to review how much your spending is being allocated for non-necessities and how frequently those non-necessities are used.

For example, fewer and fewer people all over the world are buying traditional television cable packages, meaning that many are now paying for a variety of streaming services each year, such as Hulu, Netflix, and HBO Max. If you've paid for those services before, a good way to save money would be to evaluate how many of them you actually use or how frequently you use them. If you have friends or relatives in similar or better financial situations, now would be a great time to discuss utilizing each others' streaming credentials (e.g. you pay for Netflix while your neighbor pays for Hulu, both of you have access to each account).

Other examples may come from traditional frugality when it comes to food. We understand buying take-out food because you're busy, stressed, and tired at the end of a work day, but doing it too frequently can put a considerable dent in your budget. Consider saving take-out for one special night each week or two, and instead buying cheaper frozen meals at a grocery store. In addition, when going grocery shopping, it can never hurt to try to find as many coupons or sales online or in your local newspaper in order to reduce that expenditure as much as you can.

And, if rent or your mortgage become a growing concern, we would advise having some candid conversations with your landlord or bank to see what other payment plans or discounts they may have available for the duration of the outbreak.

Now let's address concerns for the future, specifically those regarding your savings, retirement fund, and/or investments.

This may not be terribly surprising to hear, but despite the stock market's record highs at the moment, now is not a particularly safe time to invest. The rapid highs and lows brought on by the recent calamities have resulted in an incredibly volatile market, meaning that while short-term investments made at the right moment may yield huge profits, short-term and long-term investments will likely be indescribably risky. A prime example of this volatility is airline stock, which fell to record lows at the start of the epidemic, only to shoot back up during the summer when restrictions were starting to be lifted. Now, as summer comes to a close, airline stocks are due to fall yet again; while the initial bailout from multiple governments helped keep them afloat the first time, it's nigh impossible to say which ones will recover from the inevitable second collapse they will face in the near future.

In short, our advice for financial investment at the moment is to be decidedly fiscally conservative: keep or move the majority of your finances into non-invested savings accounts, and only invest money in the stock market that you are prepared to lose. If you are young and have money to spend on the stock market like it's a game at a casino, now is the time; if you have a family to care for and/or are working on a retirement fund, be safe rather than sorry.

Intuit, the financials company that owns Quickbooks and TurboTax, also strongly advises that you prepare an emergency budget aside from your regular savings in case someone in your family suddenly gets sick or laid off due to more business closings (Intuit, 2020). We endorse this view, given that the volatility of the current era suggests to us that it is better to be prepared to wait out the worst right now.

We don't think anyone should panic and throw all of their money under their mattress right now. We only advise that you remain:

- Thorough about researching what you need in your budget.

- Inquisitive about government aid programs that can help you and your family.

- Cautious about any new or high-expenditure investments until the epidemic has definitively died down.

- Careful about putting away money for the future in case anything happens to you or your family.

Chapter 8

Keeping Your Body Fit:

Methods to Ensure that You Don't Neglect Your Health

Among some of the first public spaces to be restricted or shut down at the beginning of the pandemic, the loss of the gym was felt keenly among those who went regularly. It was a consistent routine for many sharply interrupted, among the many adjustments we all had to make to our lives. Whether you were a gym enthusiast, exercised in other ways, or avoided exercise all together, one of the very important things to take care of during the pandemic is your body. The two best ways to care for your body are regularly using it for physical activity and feeding yourself well. Exercise, beyond keeping your body in shape, can also help combat the stresses of the day-to-day and keep your mind sharp. It's a great tool against the encroaching anxieties of the world, allowing you to remember there are things that you have control over.

Building an Exercise Routine

To exercise, it is generally best to have a routine that you perform at roughly the same time each day you do it and also alternating exercises. This is why many people use a gym in calmer times as it associates a place with the activity and gives them the focus they may need to not shirk their workout for the day.

Whether you have a routine built or not, it will need to be rebuilt to fit quarantine. For that reason, you'll want to consider your various options that reach beyond a dedicated gym space. Nature, in itself, is a great space for multiple cardio options, including jogging, walking, biking, and more. Narrow paths will need you to be mindful of social distancing, but this is easily done in most places. If getting outside is not particularly your idea of fun, there are multiple indoor options.

For example, there are virtually led fitness classes as well as various YouTube videos of exercise options from home experts. If you are not tech savvy, this would be a good time to reach out to your tech savvy friends and have them help you set something like this up. So it's social interaction and exercising—two birds with one stone!

If the above doesn't appeal, your other options are to think about the basics of what you can accomplish at home without an Amazon order of home-built equipment. Bodyweight exercises are a mainstay of any exercise routine, so they can be modified whatever way you like to have them work for you. Riverside Health System, in their article "Workouts you can do at home during COVID-19" recommends:

- **"Push-ups**. If you find these easy, try adding a rotation at the top of the push-up. Rotate your body so the left arm extends over your head and your body forms a T. Repeat on the other side after the next push-up. Aim for two sets of 10-12 reps.

- **Floor bridges**. Lie on your back with your knees bent and your feet flat on the floor. Push into your heels and slowly raise your hips off the ground until your knees, pelvis and shoulders are in line. You can add some difficulty by raising one leg and lowering it and repeating with the other leg. Aim for two sets of 10-12 reps.

- **Squats**. If you want to add some work for your stabilization muscles, try doing squat jumps. After doing the squat, jump up with your arms overhead. Gently land in a squat and hold the position for three seconds. Aim for eight reps.

- **Single leg balance**. Balance on one leg and slowly lift the other leg out to the side. After holding for a few seconds, lift the leg to the front and then the back. Aim for six reps before switching to the other side.

- **Lunges**. You can do traditional forward lunges or try side lunges with a balance challenge. To do this, extend your left leg to the side and bend your right leg, then push off the right leg and balance upright on your left leg with your right leg pulled up. Aim for 12 reps and then repeat on the other side.

- **Planks.** Try to hold a forearm plank or push-up position plank for 20-30 seconds. Repeat up to five times. If you find these easy, try rotating and doing side planks for the same amount of time.

- **Chair dips.** Hold on to the seat of a chair and put your feet about 18 inches away from the chair. Bend your arms and lower your hips toward the ground, then straighten your arms. Aim for 10-15 reps and repeat up to five times" (2020)

If their recommendations do not work for you, you can raise or lower the amount of reps to whatever works for your body. Creating a routine in which you warm up, stretch, and then do an assortment of these basic body-weight exercises will work to help you create a routine. Beyond these, however, there are less conventional methods of working out that will also suffice. This includes but is not limited to walking the dog, throwing a frisbee with friends or family, dancing to music, cleaning the house, and gardening. Even small exercises can ground you mentally during this pandemic.

Benefits of Exercise

But why is exercise such a vital part of dealing with the pandemic? How can staying away from or changing a sedentary lifestyle help you to combat the trials facing the world? As mentioned, there is a lot we currently cannot control in this world, especially during this frightening time.

While COVID cases are on the rise, there can be an overall feeling of helplessness that befalls us in the everyday as we consistently adjust routines and remind ourselves what is and is not safe anymore. Exercise, at the core of your being, has a profound effect on mental health and a sense of control. People who exercise regularly swear by it, not just for keeping their bodies in shape, but for its other innumerable benefits such as improving memory, relieving stress, lifting overall mood and outlook on life, and allowing you to sleep better at night.

From the Help Guide article on the subject, there are multiple studies proving that exercise helps with many mental health issue like depression, anxiety, attention-deficit hyperactivity disorder (ADHD), and post-traumatic stress disorder (PTSD) as well as general stress because it gives the bodies the chemicals it needs to fight these and many other issues as well as grounding you in the moment (Robinson, 2019). With many mental health issues being further emphasized by the shelter at home order, from feeling listless to being unable to focus or having too much time to think, a holistic approach to combating these problems will be the most effective.

Remember, though, that repeating all the benefits of exercise in your head will not automatically get you motivated to begin. Some days it can feel ridiculous or even hopeless to start worrying about your well being in this way, as if it should be the lowest on your list of priorities. If you are not naturally motivated to begin your exercise routine, you will need to examine why.

Are you giving yourself too high a bar to begin at? Are you choosing exercises that you overall cannot enjoy? Are you not allowing your rewards for completing these exercises?

Remember that exercise should not be a Herculean effort or something impossible. Any routine that has you exerting yourself far beyond your limits is too much and starting small can help you build muscles without straining them. Exercises that are hurting you are not good and should be discontinued. Not only that, it should be a mostly fun part of your day that you can look forward to.

There will always be certain parts of the exercise routine that aren't your favorite, but it can be good to give yourself a reward afterwards that you can look forward to even while completing the less-than-fun parts of your routine. If you miss a day, it's okay; just try to remember next time and move on. Despite what you may expect, it is not so much the quantity of the exercise as much as giving your body even small doses of moderate activity that will allow you to become more healthy and satisfied overall.

Takeout vs. Homemade

One of the industries that has taken many economic losses during this pandemic is dine-in food establishments. Many people are craving and missing this leisure activity, and understandably so.

While dining out is considered a treat and not always the healthiest option, the honest truth of the matter is that the difference between what you can make at home and what you can get elsewhere is knowing exactly what is going into your meal. If you have the time and can create your meals in your own space, you will have the benefit of knowing what ingredients are going in and what nutrients you are giving your body. Takeout food is not automatically unhealthy, as some might suggest, but you lose the benefit of knowing what is in it.

That being said, per the Center for Disease Control and Prevention (CDC), "there is no evidence that food is associated with spreading the virus that causes COVID-19" (CDC,

2020). Not only that, though some people may raise concerns about prepackaged foods, "there is no evidence of the virus spreading to consumers through the food or packaging that workers in these facilities may have handled" (CDC, 2020).

The real danger with food that you do not make yourself is consuming it in a place where social distancing is difficult, shared flatware or cups are being used, and the space is over maximum recommended capacity for the interior size. While being able to sit in a restaurant might allow some people to mentally find normalcy, even mitigating the risks and having outdoor dining can still lead to higher crowding than recommended.

Not only that, essential food service workers are further exposed by people dining out. For this reason, it's a good idea to take advantage of the multiple contactless takeout options provided by various food establishments.

If you do not feel up to cooking and want to put something healthy in your body, many of the sites offering contactless delivery have nutritional information beneath their menu options for your convenience. Takeout, of course, still should not be every night, even if it stimulates the economy.

Make sure to give your body the recommended amounts of fruits, vegetables, protein, sugars, and starches it needs whether you are cooking in your kitchen or letting someone else take care of your meal.

At the end of the day, we only get one body and must take care of it as best we can. While there are many different factors outside of our control, we can still control how we treat our bodies. You will need to recognize what level of exercise you are comfortable with and work at that amount to give your overall mood a boost.

Make it fun for yourself, and then fuel your body in the ways you can. Whether that is with fun rewards for exercising, or some takeout from your favorite restaurant. Your body can still thrive during this unprecedented time, so long as you remember to listen to it.

Chapter 9

DISCOVERING PATHS TO YOUR GOAL:

Uncovering Ways to Work on Your Dreams

If you've followed the tenets of the book to this point, then you have at least picked up some suggestions on how to bolster your mental health, expand your social circle, discover new modes of entertainment, maintain your relationship with the people who share your home, and improve your physical health. Despite all of this, you may still find yourself struggling with the ennui of self-isolation.

Whether you're stuck in unemployment with more free time than you know what to do with or you're in a career that you find unsatisfying, the struggles of day-to-day life from before the pandemic may still plague you now.

So what can be done to amend this?

Here's one possible path forward:

Pick a goal and go for it.

It can be something you've always wanted to do, or it can be something you've suddenly gained an interest in.

It can be personal, social, or professional.

It can be learning an instrument. It can be learning to dance.

It can be gaining a few pounds. It can be losing a few pounds.

It can be saving up a certain amount of money. It can be donating a certain amount of money to a good cause.

It can be starting up a dog grooming business. It can be starting a charity to help animal shelters.

The possibilities are endless, of course: you shouldn't feel constrained by the suggestions within this book, your personal goal is yours and yours alone.

But why, in this incredibly trying time, could it be good to pursue some sort of goal or dream? Won't that simply add more pressure to an already stressful part of your life?

Well, quite frankly, it depends. For some people who suffer from depression or anxiety, trying to force yourself to worry about yet another aspect of your life may be detrimental. If you suffer from suicidal thoughts or anxiety attacks, then we would recommend deeply searching within yourself and consulting with your physician before undertaking anything that may be too strenuous of a goal.

Otherwise, we could defer to the words of American novelist and world traveler Susan diRende:

"But you know, there is another kind of person who craves this isolation from other people and the demands of the world. No, I'm not talking about hermits. (Okay, so

hermits also fit.) I'm talking about creative people. Artists, writers, makers, inventors, entrepreneurs. These people know that they have to pull back from interaction because they need a big blank area in their heads where they can spread out the creative jigsaw puzzle and work on it without distraction. Part of the reason artists withdraw is that they know that first efforts are easily criticized and creative enthusiasm is killed. They live out the story of the Ugly Duckling, hiding themselves away and working on their vision apart from the other ducks. Because they love their inner swan.

How about you? Have you ever dreamed of doing something but put it off with "when I retire…" or "if I only had the time…" Well folks, we're all going to have the time and we're going to go stir crazy being home alone all day unless we learn from folks who've been doing it for years: writers, artists, entrepreneurs, and inventors. If you're in self-quarantine at home, instead of binge-watching or binge-reading, how about binge-creating? Time to unpack a dream. Time to see if your cockamamie contraption can work." (diRende, 2020)

In essence, to help alleviate some of the boredom and/or discomfort brought on both by this global predicament and the ennui of everyday living, it could be useful to try putting energy towards personal fulfillment, in whatever capacity you would like.

Now, most people in the world don't have any specific dream that they're working towards, aside from perhaps paying off their debt and retiring from work. This is perfectly fine! Moralizing over every individual person's measure of happiness is not our goal here.

With that in mind, now may be the time to soul search and think about things you may have once wanted and brushed off, either because the time investment was too great or because you thought it would be impractical.

While it's not comprehensive, we've compiled a list of potential goals for you to work on during quarantine. Please note that financial goals fall under our recommendations in Chapter 7.

Learning A Creative Skill (i.e. Music, Stage Magic, Painting, etc.)

Moving into adulthood, for many people, often means letting go of creative pursuits or hobbies from childhood in favor of focusing on a job or career to pay the bills. While the bills may not be any easier to pay at the moment, there is a large number of people stuck at home, and many of them have dedicated some time to teaching others about their field of creative expertise.

If you're interested in learning about music, you can purchase used instruments or songbooks for much cheaper than usual through online auction websites like eBay or Craigslist. Once you have those, there is a wide ecosystem of tutorial videos on YouTube dedicated specifically to learning about playing or performing music. There's no need to feel intimidated by this, either, because there are free lessons available for virtually every skill level, whether you had three years of experience or none at all.

The same is true for learning to do performance art, such as juggling, acting, or magic tricks, and for traditional stationary art, like drawing or wood carving. Tools for all forms of recreational art are available for use much cheaper than list price through online auction websites, and there are a litany of tutorial videos on YouTube to help you learn, regardless of your skill level.

If you're looking for people to connect with who are learning at the same rate you are, there are entire communities on forums and social media platforms dedicated to whatever niched subject you're looking to learn about. It's a great opportunity to branch out, ask questions, and learn about other people's experiences.

Learning to Speak a Language

Learning a new language can be useful to connect with older or foreign family members, expand your resume to make yourself more marketable, and make you more capable for traveling overseas. Whether it's Spanish, Chinese, French, Arabic, Latin, Afrikaans, Swahili, Gaelic, Inuktitut, or something else entirely, there are no downsides to growing your vocabulary.

Textbooks for learning foreign languages tend to come cheap whenever they're used: online auction sites for used books like eBay or AbeBooks are great providers for used textbooks from college classes at much lower prices than you would find in retail. In addition, you can also find learning software like Rosetta Stone for less than $300, which offers hours of comprehensive learning for each language.

In addition, there are millions of YouTube videos, all available for free, that will help you learn to speak virtually any language on Earth, all at a variety of different skill levels. YouTube will also allow you to practice what's called "language immersion." This means that if you're wanting to learn a language like Korean, you can spend at least an hour a day just watching videos in Korean to acclimate yourself to hearing it and understanding it.

If you're looking explicitly for people to practice your new language with, there are hobbyist forums and social media groups online exclusively dedicated to learning each language you would want to speak.

Remember: in a world that continues to be more interconnected than ever, someone who knows two or three languages is always at an advantage in the job market.

Changing Your Bodyweight/Gaining Muscle

As we described in the previous chapter, there are a variety of exercises and ways to keep in shape during this pandemic. But if you're looking to hit some specific weight goal or gain muscle mass in some specific region of your body, don't fret: there are tutorials for that, as well!

Just as is the case with all of the previous creative endeavors, there are a variety of tutorials and exercise videos available for free on YouTube that can show you how to bulk up or slim down, all for free. We would advise that you don't follow any tutorials that advise that you have to pay for some specific supplement drink, or supplement drug, or subscription-based exercise routine.

In addition, when it comes to losing weight or gaining muscle mass specifically, we advise that you remain cautious of any routine that promises too much progress in too little time—always make sure to look for secondary sources and references when undertaking anything that can affect your health. In addition, make sure all of the sources involved are properly accredited (e.g. Someone claiming that they are a medical "Doctor" who happens to have nothing but a Bachelor's in Marketing or Chemistry is probably selling you on a plan that is dangerous for your wellbeing).

Starting Your Own Business

If you're feeling the entrepreneurial spirit, then there's no time like the present for researching how to make your business happen. In a diversified, online economy like the one we have now in the 21st century, there have never been more opportunities than there are now for people to start small businesses and advertise/operate them from their computers and/or phones.

If you want to have a firm grasp of exactly what it will take to make your business work, there are countless textbooks available for cheap on eBay and AbeBooks that will help you measure out all of the potential costs for your endeavor.

In addition, we would advise that you also review some YouTube videos to get a good grasp of how to ensure that your business will be profitable, measure out the costs of running your business, make conservative and well-researched estimates for how much profit your business can be expected to make initially, and how to get your business moving on the ground.

As with the other subjects on this list, there are hobbyist forums available for starting your business.

However, we would advise that you take extreme caution in dealing with your money or your business online.

Do your research. If anyone tells you that they need money for their business OR that they're going to provide money for yours, treat it with a grain of salt and make sure to look deeply into who you're talking to. If you can't verify the identity and/or trustworthiness of the person or people you're speaking to, you should steer clear of making any financial ties with them.

Make sure that any agreements that you attempt to put in place for your money or your business are reviewed, certified, and made legally binding by a board-certified attorney.

If none of the above appeal to you, perhaps you have an idea for a special kind of home appliance or a specialized tool to help workers in difficult conditions. "Necessity is the mother of invention," and arguably, there are a lot of necessities in our society that still aren't being tended to.

So if you're interested in creating something, you're always free to look around online to make sure that someone else hasn't had the same idea. You certainly wouldn't want to work on an invention only to find that the patent already belongs to someone else.

If you've found that your idea still hasn't been implemented, then it's time to start doing some research to make it happen. YouTube will offer several tutorials about a variety of subjects (including methods for getting a patent or trademark on your idea once it's completed), but your safest bet for finding ways to be innovative and invent will likely be found in Engineering, Physics, and Chemistry textbooks. If you look around on online auction sites like eBay or AbeBooks, then you're bound to find a number of these textbooks heavily discounted.

You're also free to look through social media groups and internet forums like https://inventionideas.co/forum/ to network and discuss your idea with other inventors from around the world! Though we would also advise caution here: you don't want to give away the secrets of how your invention works or end up getting scammed by someone "collecting money for their invention."

At the end of the day, none of us can know precisely how long this pandemic will go on. All of the other chapters in this book are ultimately geared towards maintaining a certain level of safety, health, and comfort throughout this difficult period in our history.

The pursuit of a dream or goal is, ultimately, the pursuit of change. It is acting with the intent of changing something intrinsic about your life and/or the way you live it. A dream or a goal may not be for everyone—as we stated at the beginning of this chapter, if you're suffering from something like anxiety or depression, adding yet another personal responsibility into your life may not be the correct path forward for you.

There's absolutely nothing wrong with living life for the enjoyment of the everyday, seeking out the little pleasures you get from your friends, your family, your pets, and all the other things that can bring you joy.

But if you're unhappy with the routine of the everyday, perhaps it's best to take inspiration from Sebastien Chiu, a recent college graduate with a degree in film-making who helped establish a national mentorship and professional development program this summer. To quote Mr. Chiu,

"Since meeting many of our mentees and mentors, who also have big ideas but may not have the confidence, I've learned that it's just best to live by Nike. Sometimes things have to be taken by a leap of faith, and then you'll find your footing along the

way. Elaine also said it best — 'Why wait?'" (Chiu, 2020).

Chapter 10

STAYING SAFE:

For Yourself and Those Around You

We've spent a lot of time discussing ways to optimize your at-home experience, and all of those things are incredibly valuable. However, in bringing this book to its conclusion, we feel it important to emphasize what you can do to keep yourself and your loved ones safe from the virus.

At the end of the day, while keeping comfortable, financially solvent, mentally healthy, and active through the pandemic is important, the MOST important thing is to survive this, and for as many people to survive this as possible. This means that all of us have to be diligent about taking all possible precautions to avoid this virus spreading more than it already has.

The best precautions that we can all take are as follows:

I. Wear a mask when you go out in public.

II. Practice Social Distancing by avoiding large gatherings.

III. Wash your hands before you leave your home and as soon as you return home.

IV.   If you are concerned that you are showing symptoms, go for a diagnosis and push to

get tested.

Wearing a Mask

The United States Center for Disease Control (CDC) has offered this statement on

wearing a mask:

"Masks may help prevent people who have COVID-19 from spreading the virus to

others. Wearing a mask will help protect people around you, including those at

higher risk of severe illness from COVID-19 and workers who frequently come into

close contact with other people (e.g., in stores and restaurants). Masks are most

likely to reduce the spread of COVID-19 when they are widely used by people in

public settings. The spread of COVID-19 can be reduced when masks are used along

with other preventive measures, including social distancing, frequent handwashing,

and cleaning and disinfecting frequently touched surfaces.

The masks recommended here are not surgical masks or respirators. Currently,

those are critical supplies that should be reserved for healthcare workers and other

first responders. Masks are not personal protective equipment (PPE). They are not appropriate substitutes for PPE such as respirators (like N95 respirators) or medical facemasks (like surgical masks) in workplaces where respirators or facemasks are recommended or required to protect the wearer." (CDC, 2020)

So as you can read above, wearing a mask doesn't necessarily protect you from contracting the virus; rather, it protects everyone around you from catching it in the case that you have it. And if everyone around you is wearing a mask, then you are dramatically less likely to get infected. This is why there are international ordinances regarding these masks-- they are effective at preventing the spread of the virus.

We understand that some have concerns for breathing issues while wearing cloth masks, and some remain confused about how to wear them. Allow us to provide clarification on these points.

First, it is imperative to understand that if your lungs have a pre-existing issue that would cause a cloth mask to restrict your ability to breathe, then Coronavirus-19 will almost certainly devastate your respiratory system-- pre-existing respiratory conditions can effectively spell out a death sentence for the disease.

While properly created masks have been proven to be safe, even for people suffering from the breathing impairment caused by Coronavirus-19, if you find yourself unable to comfortably go in public with a mask, we strongly recommend that you *do not go in public*. You are putting yourself at grave risk. Whether it's having someone else pick up your groceries or ordering groceries for curbside pickup, or getting delivery food, or working from home, or looking into ways to get financial assistance so you can avoid going back into an unsafe work environment, if you cannot confidently wear a mask without worrying for your health, limit your exposure to the outside world as much as humanly possible.

Second, when you wear a mask, it is crucial that you cover your mouth and your nose at all times when you wear the mask. While it may be more comfortable to wear the mask below your nose, this defeats the entire point of wearing a mask-- if you sneeze and your nose isn't covered, then you've effectively spread whatever germs you may have to the air and objects all around you.

And while you are in public, it is important to keep the mask on until you return home-- eating in public should be done at a bare minimum. It is not safe at this moment in time to eat out at restaurants, even if you wear masks to go in and put the mask back on to leave. The plates and utensils within the restaurant are invariably going to be infected by you or fellow diners eating there, not to mention if someone has sneezed on any other surface while their mask is off to eat. The removal of the mask that eating necessitates means that you are endangering yourself, whoever is sitting with you, the waitstaff at the restaurant, the families of the waitstaff, and anyone who enters the restaurant after you.

The mask must remain on while you are in public, and it must remain covering the mouth and the nose. We understand that it is uncomfortable, but if you are to go in public, it's a hardship that we all have to endure.

The practices that we've been describing for the majority of this book have related directly to the practice of social distancing. If you remain unfamiliar with what Social Distancing precisely is or you simply need a refresher, allow us to explain once again.

Social Distancing is exactly what it sounds like: the practice of distancing oneself from social settings with other human beings. This means limiting contact with other people as much as is possible and, when meeting people, refraining from gathering in groups larger than 10 people and remaining at least 6 feet apart.

All of these aspects of Social Distancing, obviously, have their challenges. What if you need to go to the store or to work? What if you have to attend something like a wedding or a funeral? How do you avoid going places with more than 10 people? How can you avoid getting close to people in social settings that almost require physical closeness or intimacy?

Well, for shopping, we highly recommend ordering curbside pick-up (as many grocery stores are now offering), other forms of online shopping and delivery, or (in smaller communities) we advise being very careful to go to the store when there are less people and maintain one's distance from them physically while in the store.

As we've explained previously in this book, there are financial reasons why some may have to go into work, even if it's an unsafe environment, so it's not feasible for everyone to simply find work from home jobs or go on unemployment. In those cases, all we can advise is for all parties, workers and customers who may be interacting with them, to respect 6-foot distance boundaries and refrain from gathering in too public of places. We especially caution against going to restaurants, bars, or other places where it's necessary to eat or drink in public, at least until the pandemic is over.

As for weddings and funerals, we must also advise that such ceremonies either be postponed until after the pandemic is over or (in the cases of funerals, which almost certainly can't be put off) we advise doing video-streamed ceremonies to be followed up with grieving or celebratory meetings once the pandemic is over. Now matter how much you want your wedding to be grand, it's going to be spoiled if everyone in your family gets terminally ill afterwards. We apply this same principle in cases where you may be invited to attend something like these in person-- advise the host to postpone, and if they refuse, we advise staying home. It may create some division in your relationship, but it will be less of a divide than the one between the living and the dead.

As for settings of emotional or physical intimacy, such as movie theaters, dating spots, social clubs, and so forth, we repeat our position with regards to restaurants: refrain from attending until the pandemic is over.

Now, on the topic of schools, we understand that many schools are demanding in-person attendance of students, despite the risks we've covered already. In these cases, we advise one of three paths:

1. Enroll your child in digital schooling, at least until the pandemic is over. This may include signing up with the public or private school they attend, or it may include signing them up in an alternative online school (which you should thoroughly research the college attendance rate of before enrolling your child in, just to be certain that it is not a scam).

2. If digital schooling is not available, and you have the availability financially and the availability for time, we would advise homeschooling your child, at least until the pandemic is over. While you may not feel confident about your qualifications about providing for your child's education, this is still a much safer path forward than sending them to a potentially infectious school.

3. If neither of these are available due to your schedule and finances being strained by the pandemic, the best you can do is send your child to school with instructions to follow the 6-feet apart guideline and to wear their mask. We note that this is a last-ditch strategy, and while we acknowledge many parents may be forced to take this step, it is still less safe than having widespread digital schooling or homeschooling until the pandemic is over.

Washing Your Hands

While this aspect may seem obvious, it bears repeating: it is important to wash your hands with soap, consistently. This doesn't just mean washing your hands after using the restroom; this means:

- Washing your hands before you leave your home.

- Using sanitizer whenever possible in public spaces before and after touching surfaces or objects that have been handled by other people.

- Washing your hands or using hand sanitizer before you touch your face, especially your eyes, nose, ears, and mouth.

- Washing your hands once you return home.

- Washing your hands before and after eating food.

- ...And washing your hands after you use the restroom. We strongly urge you to continue doing this last one, too.

And while it may have been forgotten in the many months since the initial outbreak, it remains important to wash your hands thoroughly for 20 seconds at a time. This may seem cumbersome and difficult to gauge, so some people have made a variety of suggestions for songs to sing or hum while washing your hands to keep you on track and keep you from getting bored for the duration of your handwashing. Some suggestions to fill the duration at minimum include:

- The Star Spangled Banner

- Twinkle Twinkle Little Star

- "Africa" by Toto

- "Jolene" by Dolly Parton

- "Stayin' Alive" by The BeeGees

- "Love Shack" by The B52s

If You Feel Sick, Get Checked

Ultimately, this is perhaps the most important part of this book.

The symptoms of Coronavirus-19 as identified by the Center for Disease Control are, as of the writing of this book, as follows:

- Fever or chills

- Cough

- Shortness of breath or difficulty breathing

- Fatigue

- ▢   Muscle or body aches

- ▢   Headache

- ▢   New loss of taste or smell

- ▢   Sore throat

- ▢   Congestion or runny nose

- ▢   Nausea or vomiting

- ▢   Diarrhea

If you've been in public, received something into your household (such as a mailed package or delivered food) that you suspect may have been infected, or just been in contact with someone you know has the virus or may have the virus, you are at risk of having caught Coronavirus-19.

If you are experiencing any of the symptoms above in combination, then we strongly urge you to go and get tested. If you or someone you know is experiencing any of the following:

- ▢   Trouble breathing

- ▢   Persistent pain or pressure in the chest

- ▢   New confusion

☒   Inability to wake or stay awake

☒   Bluish lips or face

...Then it is urgent that you get to a hospital and get treatment as soon as possible.

In either case, we want everyone to understand that hospitals and doctors are being pressed to their limits right now as we do our best to contain this pandemic. In many cases, the physicians' first instinct may not be to test for Coronavirus, and they may insist that you probably don't need the test.

If you are at the hospital or with a physician for any of these symptoms, the common ones or the severe ones, *you have to push for the Coronavirus test.*

Do not let leave until you take the Coronavirus test.

As much as we've focused in this book on maintaining one's fiscal, social, emotional, and physical health in the wake of the pandemic, catching the disease and going untreated can be a matter of life and death. If you suspect you may have the virus by exhibiting any symptoms at all, and you have been in contact with someone or something that may have infected you, then you should get tested. It may take some pressing, as hospitals around the world are working around the clock to deal with this, but it's your responsibility as a patient to fight to get tested in the ways that you need to be. If you feel like your doctor isn't taking you seriously enough for whatever reason, it may be best to bring a friend, parent, and/or loved one whom you feel would be more confident making the doctor provide the test as needed.

If the test comes back negative, then you're in luck. Make sure to follow the rest of the practices in this chapter to stay healthy, and you're free to refer back to the rest of this book to help you figure out how to handle your wellbeing otherwise for the duration of the pandemic.

If the test comes back positive, know that you have done the brave and right thing: you checked and found that you had it before something terrible happened. From here on, trust your physician to provide you treatment-- relying on online tutorials or home remedies can be helpful for easing some daily discomfort, especially by applying some placebo comforts, but actual medicinal advice should be left to those with medical training.

And whether you have the virus or not, know that we wish you the best and we feel your struggle.

We're all in this fight against Coronavirus-19 together. If we all fight as one and follow the practices as outlined in this book to the best of our abilities, then our species has got a damn good chance of making it through.

For now, the responsibility to fight lays with each and every one of us.

We will strive to remember that as we continue our daily lives.

We encourage you to do the same.

ANNOTATED BIBLIOGRAPHY

American Library Association. (2020). Coronavirus Cases. Retrieved September 01, 2020, from https://www.worldometers.info/coronavirus/

Ashworth, B. (2020, July 4). How to Host a Virtual Watch Party. Retrieved August 15, 2020, from https://www.wired.com/story/how-to-host-a-virtual-watch-party/

Bhandari, S., MD. (2020, February 18). Stress Management: 13 Ways to Prevent & Relieve Stress. Retrieved July 01, 2020, from https://www.webmd.com/balance/stress-management/stress-management

Booking.com. (2020). Coronavirus (COVID-19) Travel Restrictions By Country. Retrieved August 28, 2020, from https://www.kayak.com/travel-restrictions

Bridges, D. (2020, March 27). The best ways to keep in touch with loved ones during the coronavirus pandemic. Retrieved July 01, 2020, from https://www.theactivetimes.com/featured/coronavirus-social-distancing-family

Brown, S. (2020, June 29). How to keep busy at home this summer. Retrieved August 10, 2020, from https://www.cnet.com/how-to/what-to-do-during-quarantine-12-fun-ideas-to-keep-you-busy-at-home-this-summer/

Center for Disease Control and Prevention (Ed.). (2020, June 12). About Cloth Face Coverings. Retrieved July 01, 2020, from https://www.cdc.gov/coronavirus/2019-ncov/prevent-getting-sick/social-distancing.html

Center for Disease Control and Prevention (Ed.). (2020, June 12). Social Distancing, Quarantine, and Isolation. Retrieved July 01, 2020, from https://www.cdc.gov/coronavirus/2019-ncov/prevent-getting-sick/social-distancing.html

Center for Disease Control and Prevention (Ed.). (2020, June 12). Mental Health and Coping During COVID-19. Retrieved July 01, 2020, from https://www.cdc.gov/coronavirus/2019-ncov/daily-life-coping/managing-stress-anxiety.html

Chiu, S. (2020, July 20). A How-To Guide Starting Your Own Passion Project in Quarantine, Learning from Our Experience. Retrieved August 25, 2020, from https://medium.com/augment-official/a-how-to-guide-starting-your-own-passion-project-in-quarantine-learning-from-experience-47e45d796acf

Consumer Financial Protection Bureau (Ed.). (2020). Protecting your finances during the coronavirus pandemic. Retrieved July 01, 2020, from https://www.consumerfinance.gov/coronavirus/

Cross, C., MD. (2020, June 04). Social Distancing: Why Keeping Your Distance Helps Keep Others Safe. Retrieved July 01, 2020, from https://www.healthychildren.org/English/health-issues/conditions/COVID-19/Pages/Social-Distancing-Why-Keeping-Your-Distance-Helps-Keep-Others-Safe.aspx

DiRende, S. (2020, March 17). Self-Quarantine: A Gift of Time to Chase Your Dream. Retrieved July 27, 2020, from https://splashmags.com/index.php/2020/03/16/self-quarantine-a-gift-of-time-to-chase-your-dream/

Intuit. (2020, May 14). 5 Tips for Managing Your Money during COVID-19. Retrieved July 01, 2020, from https://www.intuit.com/blog/financial-tips/5-tips-for-managing-your-money-during-covid-19/

Kalish, A. (2020, July 10). 14 Sites for Online Classes That'll Boost Your Skills. Retrieved June 18, 2020, from https://www.themuse.com/advice/14-best-sites-for-taking-online-classes-thatll-boost-your-skills-and-get-you-ahead

Kara, M., & Gentry, R. (2020, June 10). Working Students and New Graduates Eligible for CARES Act Unemployment Benefits. Retrieved July 19, 2020, from http://www.nasfaa.org/news-item/22188/Working_Students_and_New_Graduates_Eligible_for_CARES_Act_Unemployment_Benefits

Kassraie, A., AARP. (2020, March 23). Practical Advice for Staying Connected During the Coronavirus Outbreak. Retrieved July 01, 2020, from https://www.aarp.org/health/conditions-treatments/info-2020/staying-connected-during-coronavirus.html

Kitchener, C. (2020, March 27). How to optimize your home for self-quarantine. Retrieved July 03, 2020, from https://www.thelily.com/how-to-optimize-your-home-for-self-quarantine/

Messieh, N. (2013, January 23). 5 Sites to Discover New TV Shows You Might Have Missed Out On. Retrieved August 1, 2020, from https://www.makeuseof.com/tag/ways-to-discover-cool-tv-shows-to-watch-based-on-your-taste/

Neighmond, P. (2017, September 04). Get Off The Couch Baby Boomers, Or You May Not Be Able To Later. Retrieved August 3, 2020, from https://www.npr.org/sections/health-shots/2017/09/04/547580952/get-off-the-couch-baby-boomers-or-you-may-not-be-able-to-later

Romano, A. (2020, March 12). Stuck at Home? These 12 Famous Museums Offer Virtual Tours You Can Take on Your Couch. Retrieved July 31, 2020, from https://www.travelandleisure.com/attractions/museums-galleries/museums-with-virtual-tours

Seltman, W. (Ed.). (2019, August 17). How often should I take a break to relieve computer vision syndrome? Retrieved August 14, 2020, from https://www.webmd.com/eye-health/qa/how-often-should-i-take-a-break-to-relieve-computer-vision-syndrome

The Editors of Encyclopaedia Britannica. (2020, April 15). Black Death. Retrieved July 24, 2020, from https://www.britannica.com/event/Black-Death

The Editors of Encyclopaedia Britannica. (2020, August 27). Coronavirus. Retrieved September 01, 2020, from https://www.britannica.com/science/coronavirus-virus-group

The Editors of Encyclopaedia Britannica. (2020, June 07). Influenza pandemic of 1918–19. Retrieved June 21, 2020, from https://www.britannica.com/event/influenza-pandemic-of-1918-1919

The Editors of Encyclopaedia Britannica (2012, June 29). Pandemic status and response. Retrieved July 17, 2020, from https://www.britannica.com/event/influenza-pandemic-H1N1-of-2009/Pandemic-status-and-response

The Editors of Encyclopaedia Britannica. (2020, August 06). Plague History. Retrieved August 10, 2020, from https://www.britannica.com/science/plague/History

The Editors of Encyclopaedia Britannica. (2020, March 19). Polio through history. Retrieved June 03, 2020, from https://www.britannica.com/science/polio/Polio-through-history

World Health Organization. (2020, August). Considerations for quarantine of contacts of COVID-19 cases. Retrieved August 28, 2020, from https://www.who.int/publications/i/item/considerations-for-quarantine-of-individuals-in-the-context-of-containment-for-coronavirus-disease-(covid-19)

World Health Organization. (2020, February). Key considerations for repatriation and quarantine of travellers in relation to the outbreak of novel coronavirus 2019-nCoV. Retrieved August 23, 2020, from https://www.who.int/news-room/articles-detail/key-considerations-for-repatriation-and-quarantine-of-travellers-in-relation-to-the-outbreak-of-novel-coronavirus-2019-ncov

—